I0116440

BrainTap

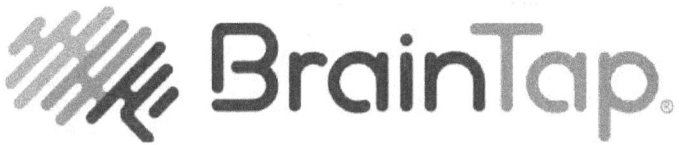

2861 Trent Road
New Bern, NC 28562
www.braintap.com

CONTENTS

Would you like to have Dr. Cidral or Dr. Porter provide a keynote, lecture or workshop on brain wellness strategies for your organization's next event? Simply call or email using the contact information provided here:

Patrick K. Porter PhD
BrainTap® Technology
1822-6 South Glenburnie Road, #362
New Bern, NC 28562
302-721-6677
patrick@portervision.com

978-1-937111-35-9

BrainTap Technologies Technical Overview Version 7.0 - January 2022.

1. Disclaimer

All research and information published herein is for informational purposes only. Readers are encouraged to confirm or verify information contained herein with other sources. The present document consists of a technical overview of BrainTap Technologies and is not in any way intended to be a complete and definite review on the matter, recognizing that the underlying information may not be current, complete or exhaustive. We strive for accuracy and completeness to support our opinions, however all information is presented "as is" without warranty of any kind – express or implied.

BrainTap Technologies does not take any responsibility and accepts no liability for any loss or damage of any kind arising out of the use, misuse, or reliance upon, the material presented herein. This work is a not intended to constitute a recommendation. Your use of any information contained herein is entirely at your own risk.

This document may contain material for the sole use of the intended recipient. Any review, copying, or distribution of this document without prior consent of BrainTap Technologies is strictly prohibited.

2. Introduction - Audio-Visual Brain Entrainment

Human brain waves, measured by an electroencephalogram (EEG), are rhythmic or repetitive patterns of neural activity in Central Nervous System (CNS) neurons. It is through these electrical signals that the brain communicates within itself and with other organ systems (Tatum 2014). Coherent and functional brainwave patterns are required for the successful processing, execution and completion of a task, whether physical (such as walking) or mental (solving an algebra problem, for instance) (Tang et al., 2016).

It is well known that brain oscillatory rhythms that fall in the 1-30Hz frequency range can be modulated or entrained[1] by an external stimulus (Thut et al., 2011). More specifically, entrainment occurs if a population of neurons in a stimulated region adopts the phase of an entraining stimulus. The entraining stimulus has two effects on population activity: (i) an increase in signal intensity (or power) as more and more neurons become phase aligned to the entraining stimulus, and (ii) phase alignment of the population activity to the entraining stimulus (Hanslmayr et al., 2019).

In healthy individuals, specific brainwave patterns are associated with various mental states. Five common brainwave frequency bands or patterns (delta, theta, alpha, beta and gamma) and related mental activities have been described (Thompson and Thompson 2003). Brainwave or Neural entrainment may provide an almost instantaneous increase in power of the stimulated oscillatory frequency (Chaieb et al., 2015), and can be achieved with minimal effort from the participant through rhythmic auditory (Isochronic tones, Binaural beats) or visual stimulation to entrain neural oscillations.

The development of Audiovisual Brain Entrainment (AVBE), also called Audio-Visual Neurostimulation (AVN), began with the observation of the effects of light in everyday life. Historically, the effect of flashing lights on humans dates back to 125 A.D., when Apuleius observed that the flickering light produced by a potter's wheel induced a

---

[1] To entrain means "to determine or modify the phase or period of something" (Merriam Webster online dictionary - https://www.merriam-webster.com).

physical response associated with epilepsy (Hutchison, 1990). Formal studies on optical stimulation by light began in the early 1900s, when French psychologist Pierre Janet observed that his patients were experiencing a reduction in psychological strain when looking at flickering lights generated by a rotating wheel spinning in front of a paraffin lamp (Tang et al., 2015). With the development of the EEG, Adrian and Matthews (1934) documented the impact of photic stimulation on brain activity. In 1949, the British neuroscientist W. Gray Walter first documented the effect of photic stimulation on both brain activity changes and subjective sensory perceptions in a study with several hundred participants. To his apparent surprise, he also found that the photic flickering stimulation evoked brain activity changes in the overall cortex and not just in the visual cortex. This observation of the "flickering phenomenon" was described in an article that has become a classic in the AVS scientific literature (Timmermann et al., 1999). Visual entrainment consists of using flashing or pulsing lights through specially designed glasses to entrain brain wave activity (Notbohm et al., 2016). Entrainment through visual stimulations such as flashing light primarily affects the primary visual cortex in occipital lobe of the brain, although, as previously mentioned, it has been shown to elicit changes in cortical activity widely distributed throughout the cortex (Timmermann et al., 1999).

Until 1960, researchers focused primarily on the influence of optical stimulation on brain activity. Beginning in 1960, a study by Gian Emilio Chatrian reported changes in brainwave voltage potential in response to auditory stimulation (clicking sounds), regardless of visual input (Chatrian et al. 1960). Then, in 1973, Oster's research on binaural beats advanced the understanding of acoustic stimulation (Oster, 1973). These are considered the beginning of auditory brain entrainment stimulation through isochronic tones and binaural beats.

Isochronic tones are consistent regular beats of a single tone (the frequency at which the tone is presented is measured in Hertz - Hz). The distinct and repetitive beat of isochronic tones produce an evoked potential, or evoked response in the brain (Radeloff et al., 2014). Frequency following response (FFR) occurs when brainwaves become entrained (synchronized) with the frequency of an isochronic beat (Pandya and Krishnan, 2004).

Binaural beats, on the other hand, represent the auditory experience of an oscillating sound that occurs when two sounds with neighboring frequencies are presented to one's left and right ear separately. This procedure produces a third phantom beat, whose frequency is equal to the difference of the two presented tones and which can be manipulated for non-invasive brain stimulation (Beauchene et al., 2016). For example, when a 400 Hz sound frequency is delivered to the left ear, while a 405 Hz is delivered to the right ear, the brain processes and interprets the two frequencies as a 5 Hz frequency. Frequency following response (FFR) occurs at the 5Hz frequency, producing brainwaves at the same rate of 5 Hz (Brain Entrainment), which can be used to "modulate" brainwave activity.

Although the exact underlying mechanisms are not well understood, audio-visual brainwave entrainment has been shown to positively affect cognition (Derner et al., 2018; Colzato et al., 2017; Hommel et al., 2016; Chaieb et al., 2015; Reedijk et al., 2013; Huang & Charyton, 2008), reduce anxiety levels (Garcia-Argibay et al., 2019; Chaieb et al., 2017; Wahbeh et al., 2007b; Padmanabhan et al., 2005; Le Scouarnec et al., 2001); affect psychomotor performance and mood (Lane et al., 1998; Wahbeh et al., 2007); improve sleep quality (Tang et al., 2015; Abeln et al., 2014); as well as induce analgesia (Ecsy et al., 2018; Ecsy et al., 2017; Tang et al., 2015) and modulate pain perception (Garcia-Argibay et al., 2019; Ecsy et al., 2017; Zampi, 2016).

3. BrainTap Research Data

3.1. Studies - Design Principles

The studies with BrainTap Technologies outlined below were conducted in accordance with the following principals:

- Pilot clinical trial,
- Randomized,
- Sample size large enough to allow for statistical significance (95% confidence interval and a *P value* ≤ 0.05).

3.2. Primary Research Outcomes

- Audio-Visual Brainwave Entrainment (ABWE) associated with transcranial Photobiomodulation (tPBM) induced statistically significant changes in brainwave activity of College Golf Players. To the best of our knowledge this is the first report to demonstrate the combined effects of ABWE and tPBM upon brainwave activity. (Study #1 - Accepted to be presented at the International Congress on Integrative Medicine and Health in Phoenix, AZ, May 2022 - ICIMH-2022).
- Audio-Visual Brainwave Entrainment (ABWE) used during daytime may be efficacious in improving chronic insomnia in adult dayworkers with normal sleep length (Study #2 - Accepted to be presented at the International Congress on Integrative Medicine and Health in Phoenix, AZ, May 2022 - ICIMH-2022).
- Audio-Visual Brainwave Entrainment (ABE) associated with Dr. Kelly Miller's "Saving your Brain" therapeutic approach positively affected Quantitative Electroencephalogram (QEEG) Analysis and Cognitive and Emotional Checklist Assessment (Study #3 -

Presented at the International Lyme and Associated Diseases Society 22nd Scientific Conference. Orlando FL, OCT 2021 - ILADS 2021).

- Although results did not achieve statistical significance when compared to baseline, ABE positively affect scores related to anxiety, general health, stress, quality of sleep, as well as work productivity and activity impairment of telemarketers. A lager sample size study is necessary to statistically confirm the effects of ABE. (Study #4 - Presented at the International Society for Neuroregulation & Research 2020 online Conference - ISNR-2020).

- Audio-Visual Brain Entrainment (ABE) significantly increased Quality of Sleep of university students (Pittsburgh Quality of Sleep Index - PQSI $p<0.05$) (Study #5 - Presented at the International Congress on Integrative Medicine and Health in Miami, FL, May 2020 (ICIMH-2020). Published at Global Advances in Health and Medicine Volume 9, 2020. DOI: 10.1177/2164956120912849).

- A single Audio-Visual Brain Entrainment session with the BrainTap Headset significantly increased heart rate variability and parasympathetic activity, as well as decreased stress index and heart rate in 100 adult volunteers. (Study #6 - Presented at the International Congress on Integrative Medicine and Health in Miami, FL, May 2020 (ICIMH-2020). Published at Global Advances in Health and Medicine Volume 9, 2020. DOI: 10.1177/2164956120912849).

- Audio-Visual Brain Entrainment with the BrainTap Headset significantly increased chakra energy levels after a single session in 100 adult volunteers (Study #7 - Presented at the Evidence based Non-invasive Therapies Conference in New Delhi, India, NOV 2019 (EBNITCON-2019).

- The Ready 4 Rapid Results H.E.A.L.T.H.Y. H.A.B.I.T.S. 13-week program did not influence quality of sleep, but positively affected Weight Loss, Mood, Anxiety, Stress. Data suggests that Braintap Brainwave Entrainment potentiated the effects of the program. Taken together, these data suggest that Braintap Brainwave Entrainment is an effective adjuvant therapy for weight loss and mood management programs. (Study #8 -

PhD Thesis in the 2022 postgraduate Program in Integrative Medicine at the Quantum University, Honolulu, HI, USA).

- Audiovisual Brainwave Entrainment positively affected Weight Reduction. Results also indicate a positive effect on stress and Heart rate variability (with increased HRV, increased parasympathetic activity and increased sympathovagal balance), although data was not statistically significant (Study #9 - PhD Thesis in the 2021 postgraduate Program in Integrative Medicine at the Quantum University, Honolulu, HI, USA).

- Brainwave Entrainment significantly decreased Stress, increased Quality of Sleep, Mood and energy levels. Actigraphy data collected with the BioStrap Bands, although not statistically significant, indicated improvement in resting heart rate, resting Heart rate variability (HRV), peripheral capillary oxygen saturation (SpO2), respiratory rate, arterial elasticity, peripheral elasticity, arterial age, sleep duration, seep efficiency (%), deep sleep , light sleep, total time Awake, sleep awakenings , sleep Score (0-100 scale), and recovery Score (0-100 scale) (Study #10 - Internal study conducted with BioStrap & BrainTap team members. Conducted in 2021).

- The combination of Brainwave Entrainment (BWE) with the BrainTap headset and compression therapy (CT) with NormaTec Pulse 2.0 Legs device effectively reduced the long-lasting or lingering symptoms of sports-related concussion in high school athletes from boys and girls soccer, boys and girls basketball, girls softball, football, and cheerleaders in comparison to Control group interventions. Better results were seen more than a year after the interventions (Study #11 - Study conducted by Dr. Arkfeld at the Gaylord High School in Gaylord, MI, United States. 2020-2021).

- Audiovisual Brainwave Entrainment potencies the effects of the Peak Performance Method (PPM). Results suggest that Braintap Brainwave Entrainment is an effective adjuvant therapy for Performance Programs. (Study #12 - Conducted with Julia Arndt (the Peak Performance Method creator - Conducted Online in 2020).

The outcomes summarized above are direct results from research conducted with the BrainTap App and/or Headset. Translation of these outcomes into consumer-based claims requires the creation of an accurate lexicon that expresses these results into meaningful and accurate representations. This is done on an individual basis.

4. Frequently Asked Questions

4.1. What is the BrainTap headset?

The BrainTap headset is on the leading-edge of the brain-based wellness approach now being advocated by health and wellness practitioners around the globe. The BrainTap headset delivers gentle pulses of light through special earphones and from within a visor. These lights synchronize with two types of sound - binaural beats and isochronic tones - to produce deep and profound relaxation and varying states of consciousness. While research has proven that both flickering light and synchronized tones can produce relaxed states, combining the two guides you to a profound level of restfulness and rejuvenation that's otherwise difficult to achieve; it is a state of tranquility that is optimum for mind/body balance, focus, and accelerated learning.

The BrainTap headset is also considered a portable achievement device. It is driven by specially encoded guided visualization audio-sessions that are uniquely encoded with Neuro-Sensory Algorithms (NSAs) to gently guide the user from the wide-awake state into a deeply relaxed optimum learning state. A minicomputer inside the BrainTap headset converts the NSA encoded signal embedded within each session, thus guiding the user through the brainwave entrainment process designed specifically for that session.

With nearly 700 sessions in more than 50 categories, the BrainTap headset system works with any smartphone or tablet that can operate Apple or Android apps.

4.2. What is brainwave entrainment?

The term entrainment refers to the synchronization of organisms to an external rhythm. In the case of BrainTap, the organism being entrained is the brain, and we do this by simulating the rhythms of specific brain wave frequencies known for deep relaxation and heightened states of consciousness.

It is the process of reaching deep levels of relaxation and then using guided visualization to form mental images. Visualization it is the primary component of the imagination and is at the core of the human ability to create, innovate and dream.

Many of history's inventors, artists and athletes attribute their success to an exceptional ability to visualize. Thomas Edison, Nikola Tesla, Henry Ford, Tiger Woods, and the great composer, Chopin, and all reported using visualization to spark their imaginations and achieve unprecedented levels of performance. In fact, Albert Einstein once said that he came up with the theory of relativity by imagining what would happen if he could travel through space on the tip of a light beam. BrainTap Technology can transport you out of a state of stress or fear, and into a new space of inner calm, peace and tranquility. A natural byproduct occurs when the body goes loose and limp, thereby creating the relaxation response - the perfect state for learning or focusing on goals.

4.3. What are brainwave frequencies?

In order to overcome the brutal effects of stress, you need to get out of the fight-or-flight response and into the relaxation response. The relaxation response can't happen as long as you generate primarily high beta brainwave activity. Your brainwave activity must dip into alpha, the intuitive mind, or theta, the inventive mind.

Many believe that theta is the optimum state for creativity and that it's the only mode in which one can make a quantum leap in consciousness. Unfortunately, theta mode is difficult to maintain. This is where the frequency following response generated through the BrainTap headset comes in; it keeps your brain engaged. By using the BrainTap headset, your brain is being trained to generate more alpha and theta waves and fewer beta waves.

4.4. What are the primary brainwave frequencies?

- BETA 13-30 Hz: This is the wide-awake alert state where you spend most of your waking life. Beta is your reactionary mind. It is the level of your mind where fears, frustrations and negative emotions are processed. This is also where your strongest filtering system operates. It is called the critical factor. The key purpose in using the BrainTap Headset is to train your mind to get out of this state where stress is dominant.

- ALPHA 8-13 Hz: This is the frequency most associated with creativity, imagination and flow. Alpha is the intuitive mind. It is also the brain state associated with relaxation, tranquility and daydreaming. Flow thinking, or a state of "inward awareness," takes place in alpha. It is also known as a super-learning state.

- THETA 4-8 Hz: This is the breakthrough state where you can reinvent your life. Theta is the inventive mind. It borders on sleep and is a meditative state with access to the other-than-conscious mind where you have higher levels of creativity, learning, and inspiration. It is also the state in which the BrainTap Headset help you to visualize and realize your goals.

- DELTA 1-4 Hz: This is deep, dreamless sleep. Delta is the unconscious mind. The BrainTap Headset is designed to keep you from falling into this state of sleep. This is why the light and sound patterns of the BrainTap Headset system continue to change throughout the session.

4.5. What is frequency following response?

Frequency following response (FFR) is the effect created through synchronized light and sound. It's how the brain "syncs" to the strobe lights, beats and tones. While your brain follows the frequencies, you experience less inner chatter and improved concentration. After a few weeks of regular use, most people gain a sense of balance and inner calm. Users report feeling serene, focused, and alert even when faced with high-pressure situations.

4.6. What are binaural beats?

These are imbedded tones that the brain naturally follows into states of deep relaxation. Within minutes your brain reaches extraordinary levels of performance that would otherwise take years of practice to achieve. Binaural beats work by tricking the brain into hearing a phantom frequency that isn't really there. For example, if we play a 220 Hz carrier tone into the left ear and a 226.5 Hz carrier tone into the right ear, your brain perceives the difference between the two, which is a subtle beat frequency of 6.5 Hz, the same frequency associated with deep, meditative states. Your brain naturally follows this frequency, and you experience this deeply relaxed state. Binaural beats are a proven self-development tool that's been researched for decades.

4.7. What are isochronic tones?

This is the newest brainwave entrainment technology. Isochronic tones are manually created, equal intensity pulses of sound separated by an interval of silence. They turn on and off rapidly, but the speed depends on the desired brain frequency. The discrete nature of isochronic tones makes them particularly easy for the brain to follow.

4.8. Why are there lights in the earphones?

The lights in the ears are set to the optimum frequency for creating a delightful feeling of serenity and balance. The earphone lights work by stimulating the ear meridians with gentle frequency pulses - so gentle that they are not visible to the human eye - to soothe, harmonize, calm and balance you.

4.9. How important are the music and tones?

The best brainwave entrainment is auditory as well as visual. Environmental sounds and music have been used for centuries in almost all cultures to create an altered state of consciousness. For example, native tribes used drums, chants, and environmental sounds like wind and rain to provide strong mental pictures and associations. There is a reason we find it relaxing to sit by the ocean and listen to waves crashing to shore or the sound of a stream as it trickles over rocks. These pleasant sounds tend to generate alpha brainwave activity naturally.

In today's frenetic culture, though, we rarely get to enjoy nature's relaxing effects. For this reason, Dr. Porter has personally encoded each session so that on a daily basis you can get a perfectly synchronized experience similar to that which nature provides. Plus, because the program is encoded into the digital audio file, you can use the BrainTap headset with any of today's high quality music players, such as the iPod or iPad, to ensure the best possible sound quality.

The music you hear on every BrainTap Technology process was composed specifically to complement the alpha/theta brainwave entrainment. The music is designed to create a full 360-degree experience that floods your mind with beautiful images and peaceful thoughts.

4.10. Why are LED's used instead of incandescent lights?

Light emitting diodes, also called LEDs, are solid-state devices that convert small amounts of safe electrical energy into light. They can be switched on and off much faster than incandescent lights, producing the crisp strobe-like pulses most effective at inducing the frequency following response needed to guide the user through the brainwave states. For BrainTap, blue LEDs were chosen for their pure, cool, calming color. Our operational research showed that users preferred the blue effect through closed eyes more than any other LEDs available. It is important to note that a person who is prone to seizures should not use the light portion of the BrainTap headset system.

4.11. Are the audio sessions effective without the Braintap headset?

Visualization and guided imagery techniques have been around for decades. These are scientifically proven modalities for behavior modification, stress relief and self-improvement. Now they are made even more effective with the added benefit of brainwave entrainment through BrainTap Technology. While there is a wide assortment of relaxation training systems, such has autogenic (self-produced) training, progressive relaxation, meditation, and biofeedback to name a few, most of these take conscious effort. With the breakthrough of the BrainTap headset, you don't have to "believe in" or "do" anything. You are immersed in the experience and don't have to create it.

4.12. Why are there sometimes two voices on the Braintap audios?

When you hear a second voice coming through one side the headphone and then other, it's not a mistake! This is a technique called "Dual Voice Processing." Dr. Porter intentionally recorded the sessions in this way to provide your brain a full holographic experience. The second voice moving from right to left and back again is there to stimulate right and left hemisphere balance. It may seem a little disconcerting at first, but don't worry, your brain will adapt quickly. The good news is, you don't have to consciously listen to any of the voices, so just relax and let it happen. The sessions that have Dual Voice Processing are marked "DV" and those that don't will be marked "SV" for single voice.

4.13. What happens during a Braintap session?

With the BrainTap Headset visor over your closed eyes and headphones over your ears, you are immersed in a perfect mixture of light and sound frequencies. Your eyes will be treated to a beautiful light show while you listen to specially designed music and the guided BrainTap Technology process. This all combines to enhance your experience and invite a higher degree of alpha/theta brainwave activity.

Some people may experience colorful geometric patterns while others may lose track of the lights completely. The light and sound pulse rate shifts from wide-awake beta to a dreamy drowsy state of theta as the session progresses. Using the science of frequency following response (FFR), your brainwave activity will follow the pulse rate of the Neuro-Sensory Algorithms. At the same time, your mind rehearses the changes or improvements you desire for your life.

4.14. What is it like to experience Braintap?

One of the best definitions of the BrainTap experience came to Dr. Porter from a satisfied client, who said, "It feels like my body fell asleep, but my mind stayed awake." This is because BrainTap generates a natural state, very much like sleep. You are then provided information that you want to apply when you are awake. This is called anchoring your vision to your timeline. It works like writing yourself a sticky note and posting it somewhere to remind you later.

Most people who want to make a change in their lives have the best intentions in the world, but the reality is, we get what we rehearse in life, not necessarily what we intend. Through BrainTap, you rehearse the new behaviors, attitudes, and beliefs you want and create in your mind a timeline for success.

During a BrainTap session, you visualize new responses to old behavioral triggers. Then, when you encounter the old triggers, you'll simply "forget to remember by remembering to forget." As your new responses take hold, you'll be convinced that you can acquire tobacco-free behaviors, think and act like a naturally thin person, or change any negative, unwanted behavior. It's that easy!

4.15. What are the benefits of using the Braintap headset?

Today, people spend thousands enhancing their bodies, but do nothing to improve the quality of their thoughts. The truth is, we can accomplish far more by managing brainwave activity and mentally rehearsing the positive, productive and healthy lifestyle we all want. Now, it couldn't be easier because the benefits of the BrainTap headset can be virtually limitless.

- Deep relaxation stimulates the production of natural, stress and tension-relieving neurotransmitters, such as endorphins.
- Helps change unwanted behaviors and habits, including those contributing to smoking and over-eating.
- Balances the brain's right and left hemispheres, inspiring both focus and creativity.
- Promotes relaxation, which contributes to maintaining healthy sleep.
- Brings more blood flow to the brain for clearer thinking and better concentration.
- Alleviates negative mind chatter and enhances motivation and performance.
- Decreases or eliminates jet lag.
- And last, but certainly not least, provides a natural ability to put stress in its place!

The majority of users report stress relief through deep relaxation, maintaining healthy sleep patterns, improved memory, improved learning skills such as concentration and recall of information, a sense of calm, increased focus, lucid dreaming, and increased physical energy.

Please be aware that while the BrainTap Headset is designed to help you reach your full potential, we cannot guarantee your results. Please understand that results will vary from person to person.

4.16. How does Braintap produce such amazing results?

The BrainTap system is designed to program behaviors so they become natural, unconscious, and automatic. You know how to drink water. You know which foods are more natural for your body. You know what exercise is. You already have these abilities. Our focus is not to give you these abilities but rather to give you a response to those abilities, thus creating responsibility. In other words, it gives you the access to the abilities you already possess! BrainTap provides the motivation, the determination, and the drive to succeed. It's a common experience that what the mind thinks about the mind brings about. The BrainTap headset is designed to help you to get into that powerful brain wave state where you can impress upon your mind the results you want in life.

4.17. How soon will I notice results?

Over 90 percent of those trying the BrainTap headset for the first time report feeling refreshed and energized right after the first process. While individual results will vary, many people report feeling more positive and motivated after just a session or two. Dr. Porter encourages everyone to listen to the full series to reap the most benefit. Those using the Habits of Naturally Thin People series may notice habit changes, such as a positive attitude about healthy foods or a desire for water, right after listening to the first process. Golfers regularly report feeling more relaxed and confident the first time out on the course after listening to Dr. Porter's Mental Coaching for Golf processes.

4.18. How will I know I've reached alpha or theta?

Everyone's experience is unique. No two people experience the same feelings or sensations while using the BrainTap headset system, and your experience will likely vary from one session to the next. You might experience lightness, heaviness, or a tingling sensation. You might even feel your eyelids flutter. You may feel as if you are drifting in and out of conscious awareness or feel dreamy, similar to how you feel right before falling asleep at night. Sometimes, as you release tension, your body might jerk or twitch. All of these are indicators that you are experiencing the alpha/theta state the BrainTap headset is designed to create.

4.19. Is it safe?

Absolutely. The only known side effects are improved memory, great sleep, focus, concentration, and reduced stress. However, flashing lights have been known to cause problems in people who suffer from serious medical conditions like epilepsy, seizure disorders, brain injury, or photosensitivity. If you have any of these concerns, you should ask your medical professional if light and sound technology is right for you.

4.20. Who can benefit from Braintap technology?

Anyone who is not sensitive to flashing light can benefit from BrainTap technology. The BrainTap Headset, used in combination with the guided visualization audio-sessions creates a potent tool for creating laser-like focus and enhanced performance.

The light intensity on the BrainTap Headset is adjustable, so those who have minor light sensitivity can almost always find a setting that's right for them. Those diagnosed with light sensitivity seizures should not use the flashing lights in the visor, but can experience the profound benefits of the guided visualization, auriculotherapy and relaxing tones.

4.21. Can everyone use the Braintap headset?

Generally speaking, any person can achieve alpha/theta brainwave states and can benefit from BrainTap Technology. However, the sessions are recommended for persons with a healthy brain. Persons with severe mental disorders should not use the BrainTap

Headset. Flashing lights have been known to trigger seizures in certain cases. While this disorder is rare, people who have a seizure disorder of any kind should not use the lights in the visor. These people can still benefit without the lights. If you are unsure, ask your doctor before proceeding.

4.22. Can children use the Braintap headset?

As long as the child can sit still in a chair for 10 or 20 minutes, the BrainTap headset can be of benefit, and there are a variety of sessions geared toward children, tweens and young adults. We have children as young as five years old using the technology before bed and getting great results. The "Accelerated Learning Series" can be used by teens and adults alike.

5. Studies

5.1. Abstracts from conferences

5.1.1. Study #1. Accepted to be presented at the International Congress on Integrative Medicine and Health in Phoenix, AZ, May 2022 - ICIMH-2022.

Title

Effect of Brainwave Entrainment and Transcranial Photobiomodulation on Brainwave Power of College Golf Players.

Authors

Francisco Jose Cidral-Filho, Ph.D.[1], Eber Fontes, Esp.[2], Patrick Porter, Ph.D.[2], Geraldine Perez, Ph.D.[3]

1. Laboratory of Experimental Neurosciences. University of Southern Santa Catarina, SC, Brazil.
2. Physical therapy Program. University of Ribeirao Preto, SP, Brazil.
3. Postgraduate Program in Integrative Medicine. Quantum University. Honolulu, HI, USA.
4. Disability Support Services. Seminole State College of Florida. Sanford/Lake Mary Campus. Sanford, FL, USA.

Background

Transcranial photobiomodulation (tPBM) is a novel form of neuromodulation, based on non-retinal exposure to light at specific wavelengths, mainly in the red or near-infrared range. tPBM has been shown to improve memory, attention, and induce sleep regulation. Brainwave entrainment (BWE) refers to the use of rhythmic stimuli with the intention of producing a frequency-following response of brainwaves to match the frequency of the stimuli. The stimulus is usually either visual (flashing lights) or auditory (pulsating tones). BWE has been shown to influence Brainwave power and significantly improve attention; as well as Reduce anxiety and stress. The combination of tPBM and BWE has not yet been studied.

Objective

Investigate the effect of Brainwave Entrainment and Transcranial Photobiomodulation on Brainwave Power of College Golf Players.

Methods

Trial was pre-approved by Seminole State College Internal Review Board. Participants were screened and asked to sign an Informed Consent Form. Sample size consisted of 8 adult female College Golf Athletes (Average of 18 years of age) with no hearing disabilities and no prior use of BWE or tPBM. Participants were randomly assigned by simple draw to either Group A or B. Group A underwent BWE sessions 2 times a week for the first 3 weeks, then tPBM 2 times a week for the next 3 weeks; Group B underwent tPBM for the first 3 weeks, then BWE for the next 3, totaling a 6-week intervention period. BWE was delivered in 20-minute sessions with a BrainTap headset (New Bern, NC). BWE Sessions consisted of Binaural beats and Isochronic Tones varying from 18 to 0.5 HZ as well as visual Entrainment through light-emitting diode lights at 470 nanometers (nm) flickering at the same rate (18 to 0.5 HZ). tPBM was delivered in 10-minute sessions with a tPBM helmet composed of 660 nm (n=100) and 850nm (n=100) evenly distributed. Total irradiance delivered per session was 1000 mW/cm2 per minute. Evaluation of total brainwave power was conducted with the Emotiv Epoc+ 14-Channel Wireless electroencephalogram (EEG) Headset (San Francisco, CA). EEG sessions were conducted at baseline and after 6 weeks and consisted of 2-minute eyes open immediately followed by 2-minute eyes closed readings. The average of the overall brainwave power of the 14 channels is reported.

Results

Two-tailed Paired T-test with 95% confidence interval (GraphPad software v.9, La Joula, CA) between baseline and end of study EEG evaluations demonstrated the following: decrease in Gamma (-46%, $p<0.0098$), Low Beta (-24.4%, $p<0.1171$), High Beta (-46%, $p<0.0278$), and Theta (-42%, $p<0.3206$); and an increase in Alpha (90%, $p<0.0009$).

Conclusion

The interventions used herein induced statistically significant changes in brainwave activity of College Golf Players. To the best of our knowledge this is the first report to demonstrate the combined effects of BWE and tPBM upon brainwave activity.

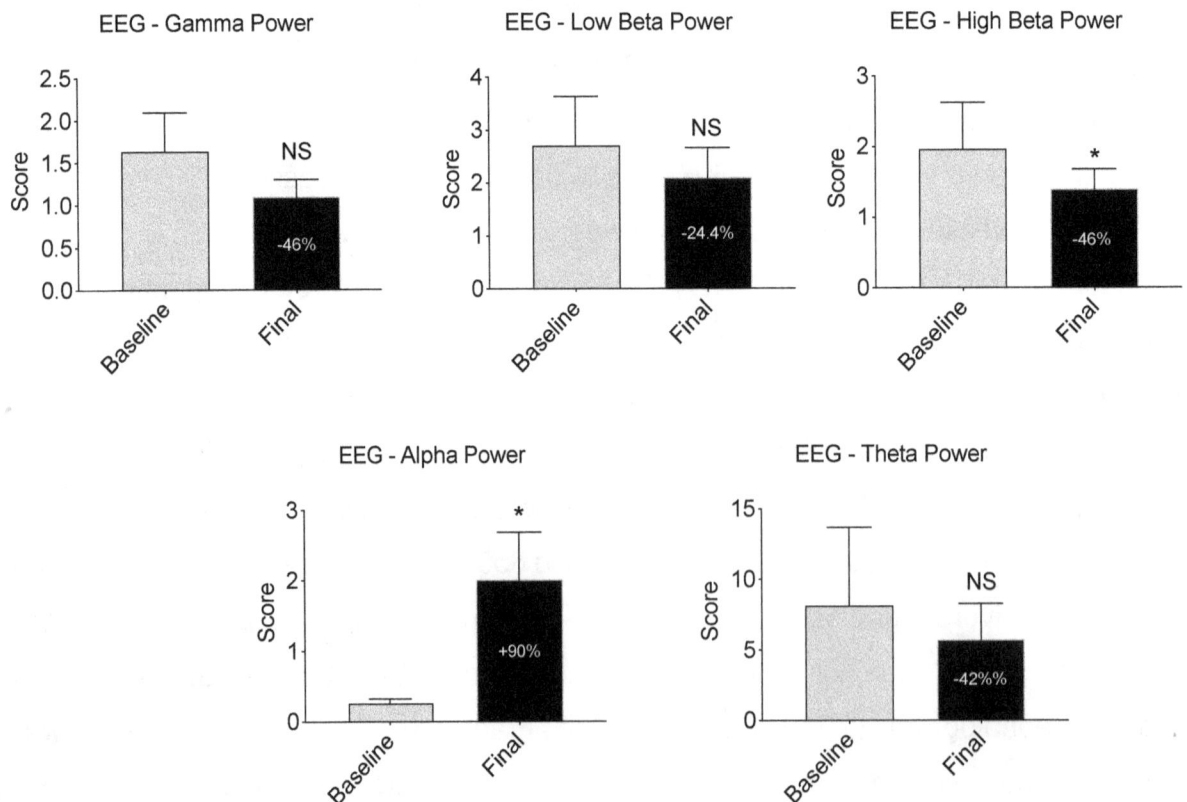

Figure 1 - The effect of Brainwave Entrainment and Transcranial Photobiomodulation on Brainwave Power of College Golf Players. NS = Not statistically significant. *p<0.05 (paired T-Test 95% with a confidence interval - Graphpad Prism software, USA).

- www.braintap.com
- 2861 Trent Road
- New Bern, NC 28562

BrainTap

5.1.2. Study #2. Accepted to be presented at the International Congress on Integrative Medicine and Health in Phoenix, AZ, May 2022 - ICIMH-2022.

Title

Use of open-loop audio-visual entrainment to Improve Chronic Insomnia in Adult Dayworkers with Normal Sleep Duration.

Authors

Michael Keown, Ph.D. Student[1], Francisco Jose Cidral-Filho, Ph.D.[2], Patrick Porter, Ph.D.[1]

1. Postgraduate Program in Integrative Medicine. Quantum University. Honolulu, HI, USA.
2. Laboratory of Experimental Neurosciences. University of Southern Santa Catarina, SC, Brazil.

Background

Chronic primary insomnia is one of the most common sleep disorders among adults, including day workers, and is characterised by difficulties initiating (latency) and/or maintaining sleep as well as early morning awakening, which can result in daytime impairment. Aside from conventional pharmacotherapeutic and non-pharmacotherapeutic treatment, no complementary intervention has been found to treat chronic 'primary' insomniac adults with normal sleep duration (> 6h). Previous studies have found that open-loop audio-visual entrainment (OLAVE) potentially reduces excessive hyperarousal that is thought to contribute to difficulties with impairment at daytime and initiating and maintaining sleep at nighttime.

Objective

The goal of this study was to assess the efficacy of open-loop audio-visual entrainment to improve chronic insomnia in adult dayworkers with normal sleep duration.

Methods

Fifteen middle-aged day workers were randomly assigned to one of two intervention groups: OLAVE (n = 8, with the Braintap Headset - New Bern, NC) or CONTROL (n = 7) (placebo group) for a period of 6 weeks. Both groups attended six, weekly sessions, during the day, at the same time and day of the week. During the 10-week trial, participants completed four different questionnaires including three self-assessment questionnaires for insomnia symptoms, sleep quality and emotional impairment, and a sleep diary. Actigraph, heart rate and heart rate variability readings were also recorded during the intervention.

Results

After 6 weeks, between-group differences were found in sleep fragmentation (Wake After Sleep Onset - WASO, $p=0.04$) and sleep quality (Pittsburgh Quality of Sleep index - PSQI, $p<0.0001$; Consensus Sleep Diary - CSD, Total Sleep Time Subset, $p=0.004$) in the OLAVE group. Within-group differences showed that both groups reported some improvement in sympathovagal balance and significant improvements in insomnia symptoms (Insomnia Severity Index - ISI, $p<0.05$) and emotional reactivity (impairment) ($p<0.05$), which continued to the end of the trial. Improvement in sleep quality (PSQI, $p<0.001$, CSD, $p<0.01$), WASO ($p<0.01$) and sleep efficiency ($p<0.05$) in the OLAVE group were reported at the 2-week post-intervention period.

Conclusion

Results suggest that OLAVE technology used during daytime may be efficacious in improving chronic insomnia in adult dayworkers with normal sleep length. Further exploration of OLAVE as a non-pharmacotherapeutic intervention for reducing chronic insomnia in adult dayworkers is warranted.

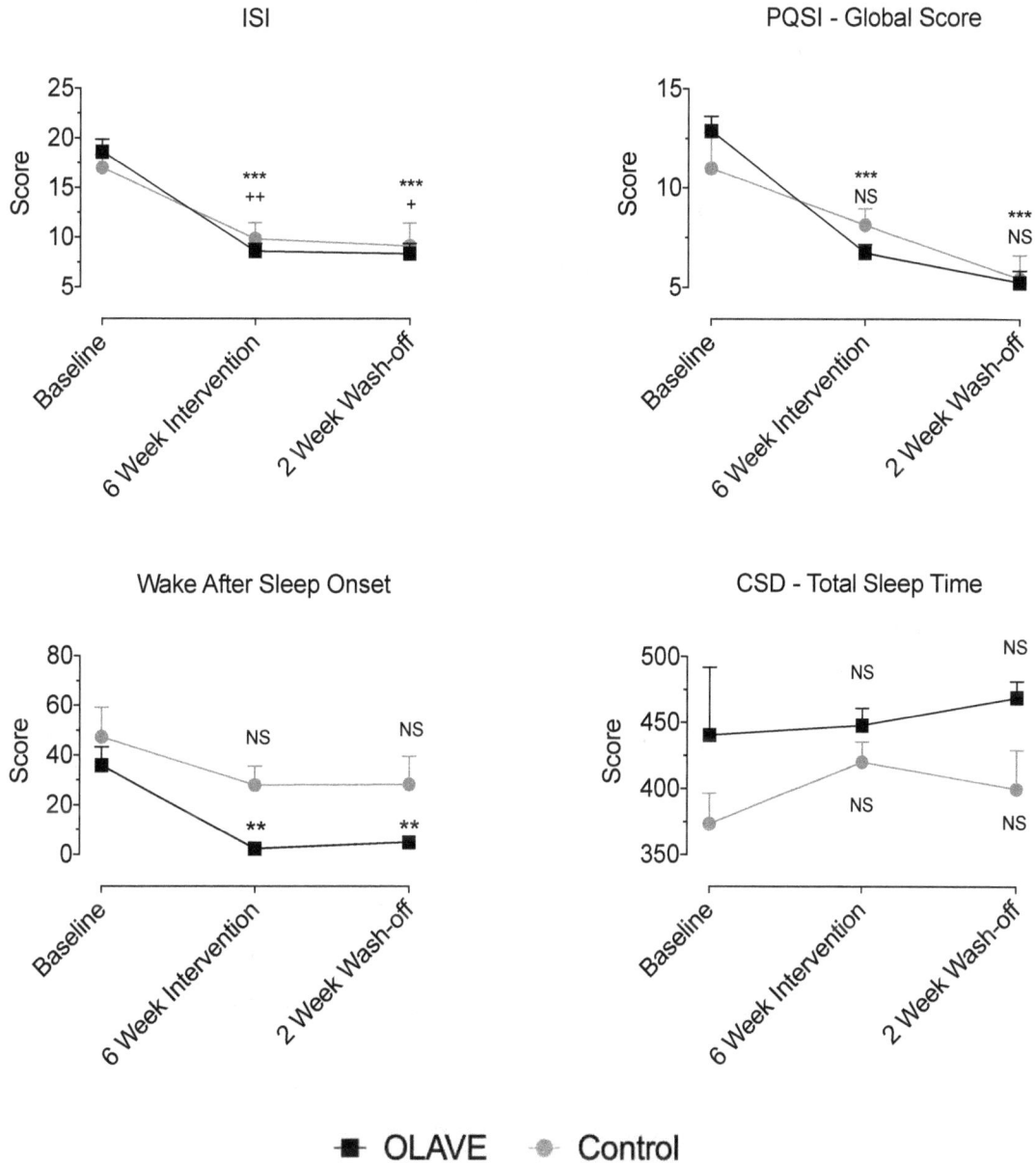

Figure 1 - The use of open-loop audio-visual entrainment to Improve Chronic Insomnia in Adult Dayworkers with Normal Sleep Duration. Effects upon Insomnia Severity Index (ISI), WASO (Wake After Sleep Onset), Pittsburgh Quality of Sleep index (PSQI), Consensus Sleep Diary (CSD, Total Sleep Time Subset). When comparing within-group differences with Baseline: NS = Not statistically significant, **p<0.01, ***p<0.001 for OLAVE group; +p<0.05, ++p<0.01 for Control Group (Two-way ANOVA repeated measures followed by Bonferroni post-hoc Test - Graphpad Prism software, USA).

5.1.3. Study #3. Presented at the International Lyme and Associated Diseases Society 22nd Scientific Conference. Orlando FL, OCT 2021 - ILADS 2021.

Title

Audiovisual Brain Entrainment associated with "Saving your Brain" therapeutic approach on Quantitative Electroencephalogram Analysis and Cognitive and Emotional Checklist Assessment.

Authors

Cidral-Filho, F.J.[1]; Porter, P.[2], Miller, K[2].

Affiliations

1. Laboratory of Experimental Neurosciences. University of Southern Santa Catarina, SC, Brazil.
2. Postgraduate Program in Integrative Medicine. Quantum University. Honolulu, HI, USA.

Objective

The objective of this study was to investigate the effect of Audio-Visual Brainwave Entrainment (ABE) associated with "Saving your Brain" therapeutic approach on Quantitative Electroencephalogram (QEEG) Analysis and the Cognitive and Emotional Checklist Assessment.

Methods

Participants (n=6, 5 female, 1 male, average of 61.3 years old) underwent approximately 6 weeks of therapy, i.e., three daily ABE sessions with the BrainTap headset (New Bern - NC - USA) associated with "Saving your Brain" therapeutic approach. The study was conducted at Dr. Kelly Miller's Clinic, Tampa, FL - USA and data analyses at the Experimental Neuroscience Laboratory (LANEX) of the University of Southern Santa Catarina - Brazil. QEEG Analysis was conducted with the NewMind QEEG Analysis and

Client Management system (NewMind, USA) at baseline and after ~3 weeks of intervention.

Results

In comparison to baseline evaluation, the therapeutic approach used herein effectively decreased Metabolic Score (44.94%, data not statically significant - NS) and Total response time (7.97%, NS) (Figure 1A and B, respectively); as well as increased brain plasticity (45.8%), normalization (46.8%), and reorganization (42.8%) (Figure 2). Additionally, cognitive and emotional checklist assessment indicate positive effects on Attention (16.6%, NS), Memory (22.31%, $p<0.05$), Depression (62.05%, $p<0.05$), and Anxiety (31.77%, NS) (Figure 3A to D, respectively).

Conclusion

Audio-Visual Brainwave Entrainment (ABE) associated with Dr. Kelly Miller's "Saving your Brain" therapeutic approach positively affected Quantitative Electroencephalogram (QEEG) Analysis and Cognitive and Emotional Checklist Assessment.

Limitations

Small sample size (n=6).

A   Metabolic Score

B   Response Time

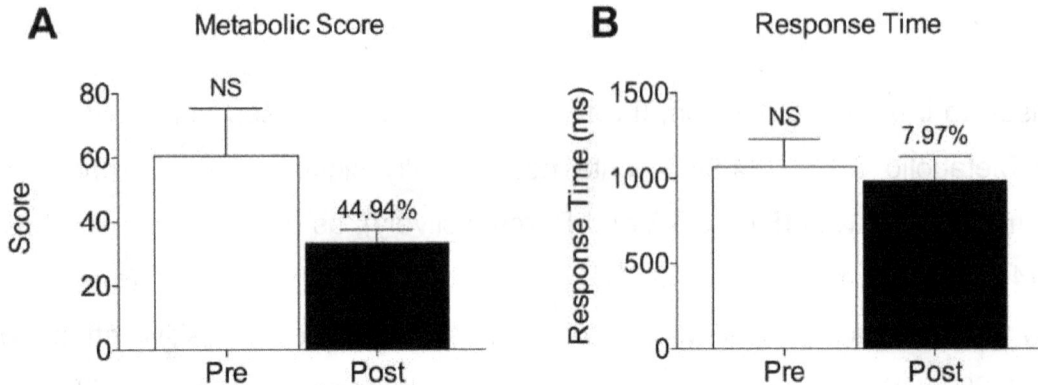

*Lower scores indicate more favorable results

Figure 1 - Effect of Audiovisual Brain Entrainment associated with Dr. Kelly Miller's "Saving your Brain" therapeutic approach on (A) Metabolic score and (B) response time. NS = Not statistically significant (paired T-Test 95% confidence interval - Graphpad Prism software, USA).

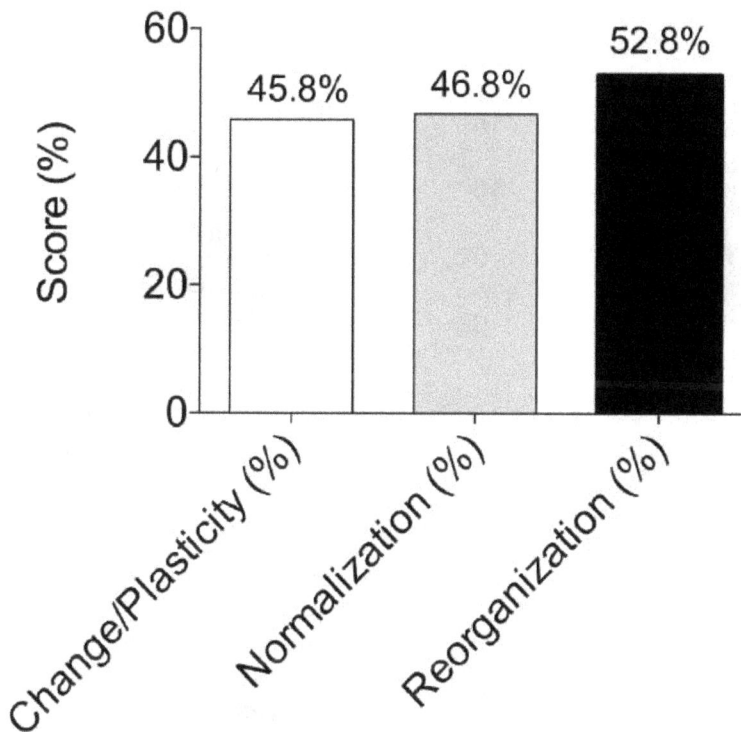

Figure 2 - Effect of Audiovisual Brain Entrainment associated with Dr. Kelly Miller's "Saving your Brain" therapeutic approach on Quantitative Electroencephalogram Analysis (NewMind QEEG Analysis and Client Management system - NewMind, USA)

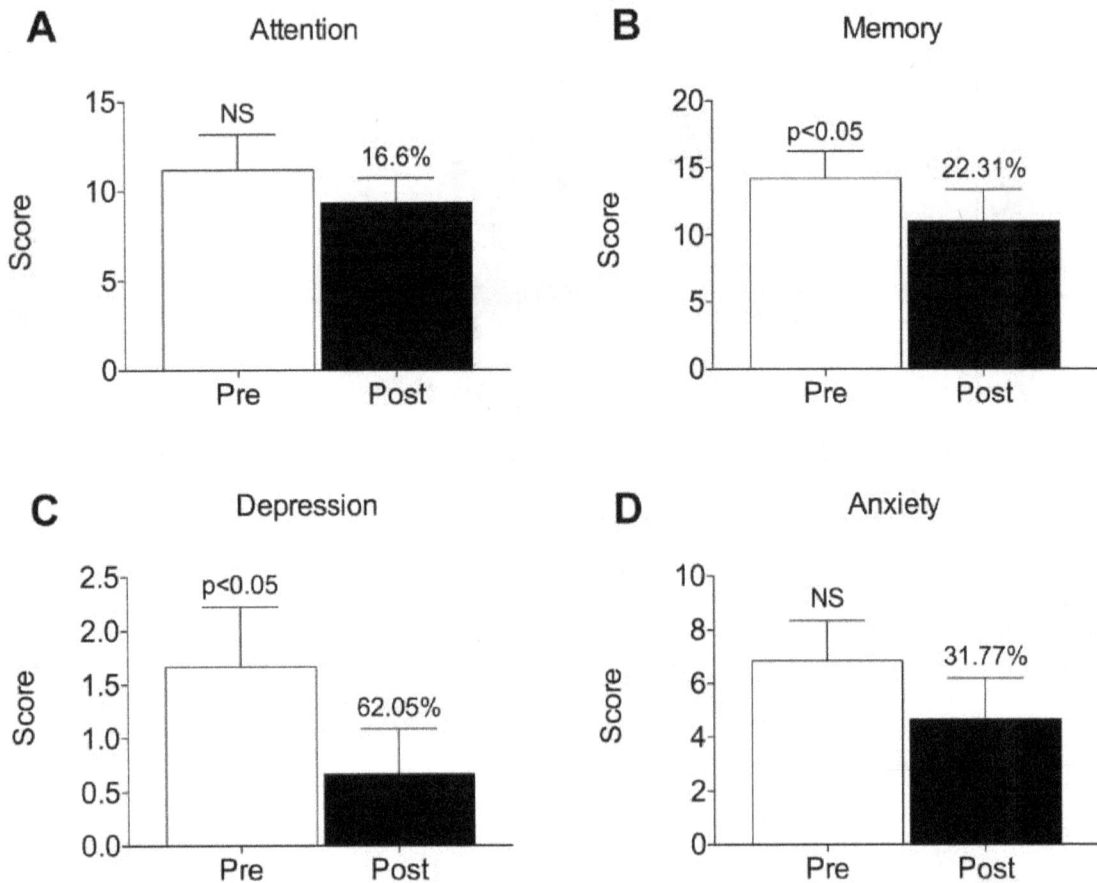

A Attention
B Memory
C Depression
D Anxiety

*Lower scores indicate more favorable results

Figure 3 - Effect of Audiovisual Brain Entrainment associated with Dr. Kelly Miller's "Saving your Brain" therapeutic approach on the Cognitive and Emotional Checklist Assessment (A) Attention Score, (B) Memory Score, (C) Depression Score, and (D) Anxiety Score. p<0.05 when comparing to baseline to post-intervention. NS means NS = Not statistically significant (paired T-Test 95% confidence interval - Graphpad Prism software, USA).

5.1.4. Study #4. Presented at the International Society for Neuroregulation & Research 2020 online Conference - ISNR-2020.

Title

Effect of Audio-Visual Brain Entrainment on Mood, Sleep and Work Productivity of Professional Telemarketers.

Authors

Francisco J Cidral-Filho[1], Patrick K Porter[2], Rodolfo B Parreira[3,4,5], Noemy Ferreira de Castro[3], Maria Luisa Ramos Mendes[3], Afonso Salgado[3,4]

1. Laboratory of Experimental Neurosciences. University of Southern Santa Catarina, SC, Brazil.
2. Postgraduate Program in Integrative Medicine. Quantum University. Honolulu, HI, USA.
3. Residence Program in Manipulative, Complementary and Integrative Physical Therapy, Philadelphia University Center, PR, Brazil.
4. PostureLab, Paris France.
5. Health Sciences Program, Santa Casa de São Paulo School of Medical Sciences, SP, Brazil.

Background

Audio Visual Brainwave entrainment (ABE) occurs when brainwaves synchronize to external rhythmic stimuli, e.g, visual (flickering lights), auditory (Isochronic tones, and/or Binaural beats) or physical (physical vibration).

Objective

The objective of this study was to investigate the effect of the Audio-Visual Brain Entrainment (ABE) on Anxiety, General Health, Stress, Quality of Sleep and Work productivity and Activity Impairment of telemarketers.

Methods

The study was conducted at the Salgado Institute of Integrative Health, Londrina, PR - Brazil, and the protocol was approved by the Institutions Ethics Committee. Sample size consisted of 13 telemarketers (3 males and 10 females). ABE was delivered with a BrainTap headset (New Bern - NC - USA) in 20-minute sessions 3 times a week for 6 weeks. Session consists of Binaural beats (18 to 0.5 HZ), Isochronic Tones (18 to 0.5 HZ) and visual Entrainment (470 nanometers LEDs flickering at 18 to 0.5 HZ). The following questionnaires were applied at baseline and after 6 weeks: The Hamilton Anxiety Rating Scale (HAM-A) that measures the severity of anxiety symptoms; the General Health Questionnaire (GHQ-12), a screening device for identifying minor psychiatric disorders; the Perceived Stress Scale (PSS-10), the most widely used psychological instrument for measuring the perception of stress; the Pittsburgh Quality of Sleep Index (PQSI), that scores sleep quality; and the Work Productivity and Activity Impairment Questionnaire (WPAI), that measures impairments in work and activities.

Results

ABE positively affected all scores: HAM-A (22.95%); GHQ-12 (10.93%); PSS-10 (16.86%); PQSI (14.51%); as well as WPAI (absenteeism, 41.66%; presenteeism, 56.25%; work productivity, 56.22%; and activity Impairment due to health, 76%).

Conclusion

Although results did not achieve statistical significant when compared to baseline, ABE positively affect scores related to anxiety, general health, stress, quality of sleep, as well as work productivity and activity impairment of telemarketers. A lager sample size study is necessary to statistically confirm the effects of ABE.

BrainTap

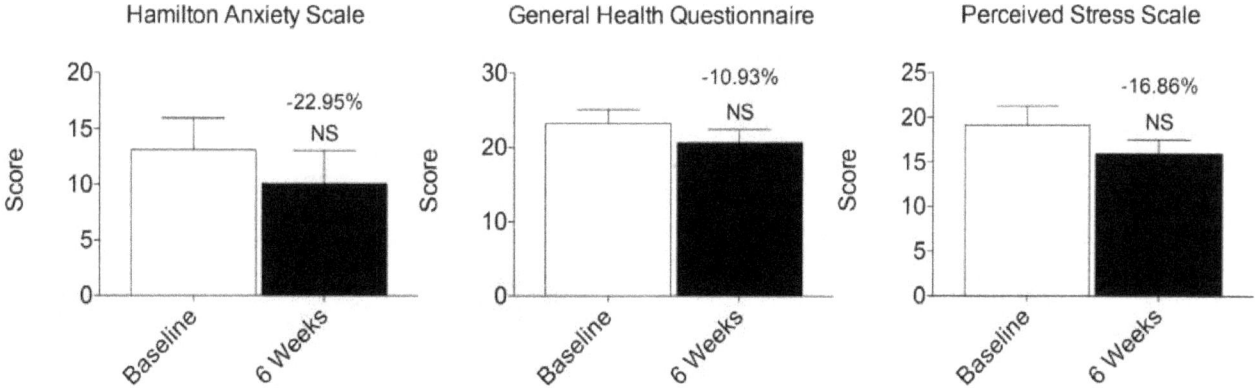

Figure 1 - The Effect of Audio-Visual Brain Entrainment on the Hamilton Anxiety Rating Scale (HAM-A), the General Health Questionnaire (GHQ-12), and the Perceived Stress Scale (PSS-10). NS: Not statistically significant (Paired T-Test with a 95% with a confidence interval - Graphpad Prism software, v.8, La Jolla, CA, USA).

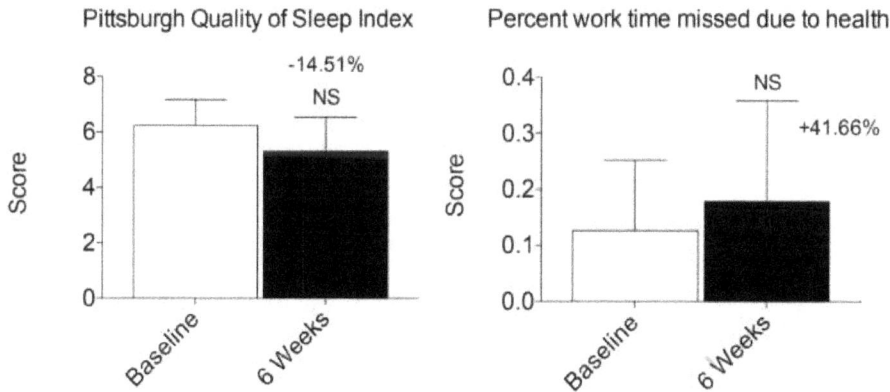

Figure 2 - The Effect of Audio-Visual Brain Entrainment on the Pittsburgh Quality of Sleep Index (PQSI), and the Work Productivity and Activity Impairment Questionnaire (WPAI). NS: Not statistically significant (Paired T-Test with a 95% with a confidence interval - Graphpad Prism software, v.8, La Jolla, CA, USA).

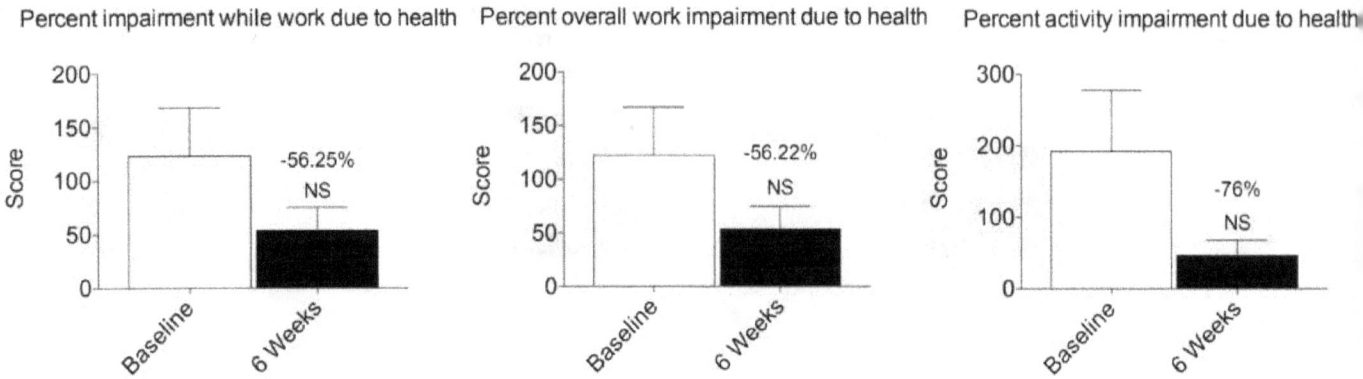

Figure 3 - The Effect of Audio-Visual Brain Entrainment on the Work Productivity and Activity Impairment Questionnaire (WPAI). NS: Not statistically significant (Paired T-Test with a 95% with a confidence interval - Graphpad Prism software, v.8, La Jolla, CA, USA).

5.1.5. Study #5. Presented at the International Congress on Integrative Medicine and Health in Miami, FL, May 2020 (ICIMH-2020). Published at Global Advances in Health and Medicine Volume 9, 2020. DOI: 10.1177/2164956120912849.

Title

Effect of Audio-Visual Brain Entrainment on Mood and Quality of Sleep: a pilot trial with university students.

Authors

Daiana Cristina Salm[1,2], Luiz Augusto Belmonte[1,2], Bruna Hoffmann de Oliveira[1,2], Luana Meneghini Belmonte[1,2], Francisco J Cidral-Filho[1,2], Patrick Porter[3] and Daniel Fernandes Martins[1,2]

1. Experimental Neuroscience Laboratory (LaNEx), University of Southern Santa Catarina, SC, Brazil.
2. Postgraduate Program in Health Sciences, University of Southern Santa Catarina, SC, Brazil.
3. Postgraduate Program in Integrative Medicine. Quantum University. Honolulu, HI, USA.

Objective

The Study Objective was to investigate the effect of the Audio-Visual Brain Entrainment (ABE) on Mood and Quality of Sleep of university students.

Methods

The study was conducted at the Laboratory of Experimental Neuroscience - University of Southern Santa Catarina (UNISUL), Brazil, and the protocol was approved by the Institutions Ethics committee. Informed consent forms were obtained during patient screening phase of the study at the site of the tests.

Sample size consisted of 7 university students (Four males and three females. Ages between 20 and 58), who were not making use of analgesics, anti-inflammatories or sleep aids 7 (seven) days prior to, as well as during the study, and who had no hearing disabilities. ABE was delivered with a BrainTap headset (New Bern - NC – USA; Figure 1, A & B) in 20-minute sessions 3 times a week for 6 weeks. Session consists of Binaural beats at 18 to 0.5 HZ, Isochronic Tones at 18 to .0.5 HZ and visual Entrainment through light- emitting diode lights at 470 nanometers (nm) flickering at 18 to 0.5 HZ. The following questionnaires were applied at baseline and after 6 weeks: Epworth Sleepiness Scale - Daytime sleepiness (ESS), Insomnia Severity Index (ISI), Pittsburgh Quality of Sleep Index (PQSI), Depression Anxiety and Stress Scale (DASS-21), and Perceived Stress Scale (EPS-10).

Results

ABE effectively reduced ISI (data not statistically significant); PQSI ($p<0.05$); DASS-21 (data not statistically significant); and EPS-10 (data not statistically significant). The participants reported feeling very relaxed during the sessions.

Conclusion

Despite the reduced sample size (n=7), results indicate that Audio-Visual Brain Entrainment (ABE) significantly increased Quality of Sleep of university students (PQSI $p<0.05$). A lager sample size study is necessary to confirm and extend the effects of ABE on Mood.

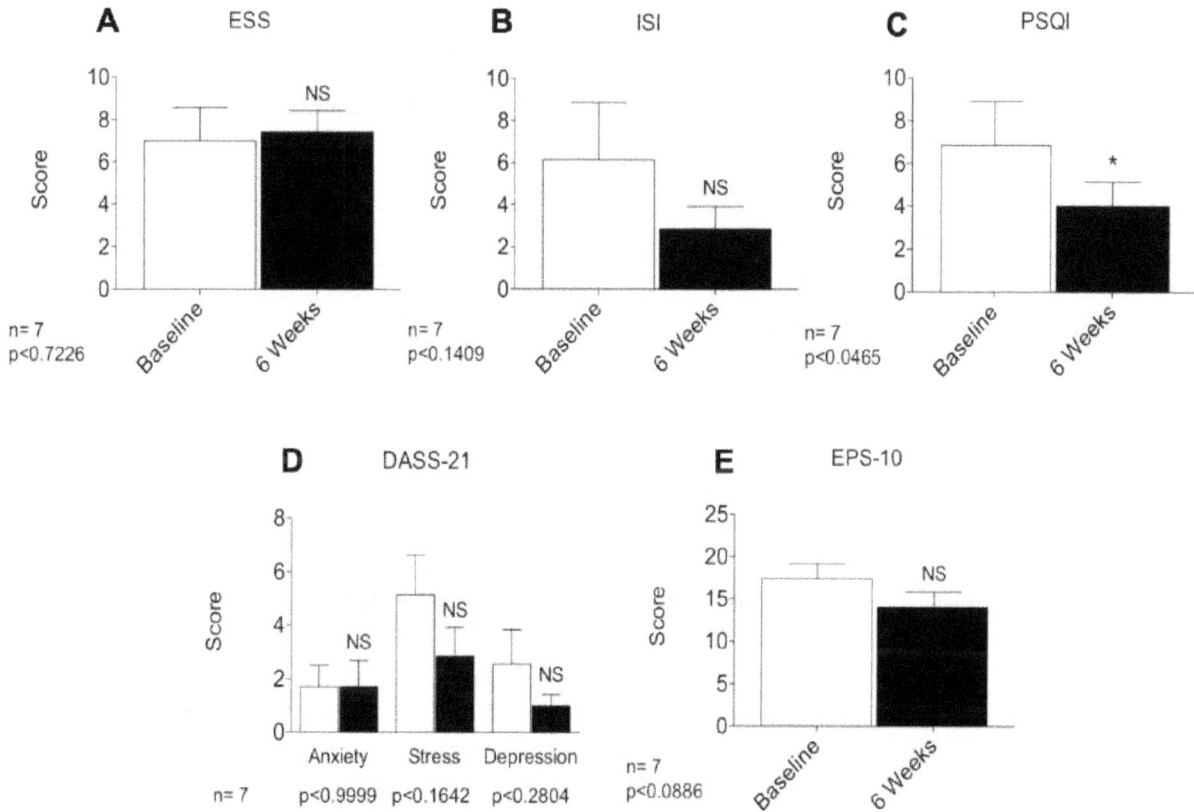

Figure 1 - Effect of Audio-Visual Brain Entrainment on Mood and Quality of Sleep. A) Epworth Sleepiness Scale; B) Insomnia Severity Index; C) Pittsburgh Quality of Sleep Index; D) Depression Anxiety and Stress Scale; E) Perceived Stress Scale. Data were expressed as mean ± standard deviation (SD) n = 7. Student's T-test was used. *p<0.05 when compared with baseline evaluation. NS: not statistically significant.

5.1.6. Study #6. Presented at the International Congress on Integrative Medicine and Health in Miami, FL, May 2020 (ICIMH-2020). Published at Global Advances in Health and Medicine Volume 9, 2020. DOI: 10.1177/2164956120912849.

Title

Effect of a single Audio-Visual Brain Entrainment session on Heart Rate Variability: a clinical trial with 100 adult volunteers.

Authors

Michael Porter[1], Patrick Porter[1,2], Francisco J Cidral-Filho[1]

1. Laboratory of Experimental Neurosciences. University of Southern Santa Catarina, SC, Brazil.
2. Postgraduate Program in Integrative Medicine. Quantum University. Honolulu, HI, USA.

Objective

The objective of this study was to investigate the effect of the Audio-Visual Brain Entrainment (ABE) on Heart Rate Variability.

Methods

Sample size consisted of 100 adult volunteers (50 males and 50 females) with no hearing disabilities. ABE was delivered with a BrainTap headset (New Bern - NC - USA) in a 20-minute session. Session consists of Binaural beats at 18 to 0.5 HZ, Isochronic Tones at 18 to .0.5 HZ and visual Entrainment through light-emitting diode lights at 470 nanometers (nm) flickering at 18 to 0.5 HZ. Heart rate Variability (Dinamika HRV - Advanced Heart Rate Variability Test System, Moscow, Russia) was assessed at baseline and after ABE session.

Results

ABE significantly (1) increased Heart Rate Variability: HRV Index (A low HRV is associated with an increased risk of cardiovascular disease - $p<0.001$, 21.8%) and RRNN (RR normal-to-normal intervals; a marker of overall HRV activity - $p<0.001$, 6.8%); (2) increased Parasympathetic activity markers: RMSSD (Root Mean Square of the Successive RR interval Differences - $p<0.0001$, 32.2%), NN50 (The number of pairs of successive NN (R-R) intervals that differ by more than 50 ms - $p<0.0001$, 50.6%), pNN50% (The proportion of NN50 divided by the total number of NN (R-R) intervals - $p<0.001$, 51.6%), HFnu (High Frequency Band: index of modulation of the parasympathetic branch of the autonomic nervous system - $p<0.0336$, 37.1%), and LFnu: (Low Frequency Band: general indicator of aggregate modulation of both the sympathetic and parasympathetic branches of the Autonomic Nervous System - $p<0.0048$, 45.1%); and (3) decreased Stress Index ($p<0.001$, 38.4%) and Heart Rate ($p<0.0001$, 6.2%).

Conclusion

A single Audio-Visual Brain Entrainment session with the BrainTap Headset significantly increased heart rate variability and parasympathetic activity, as well as decreased stress index and heart rate.

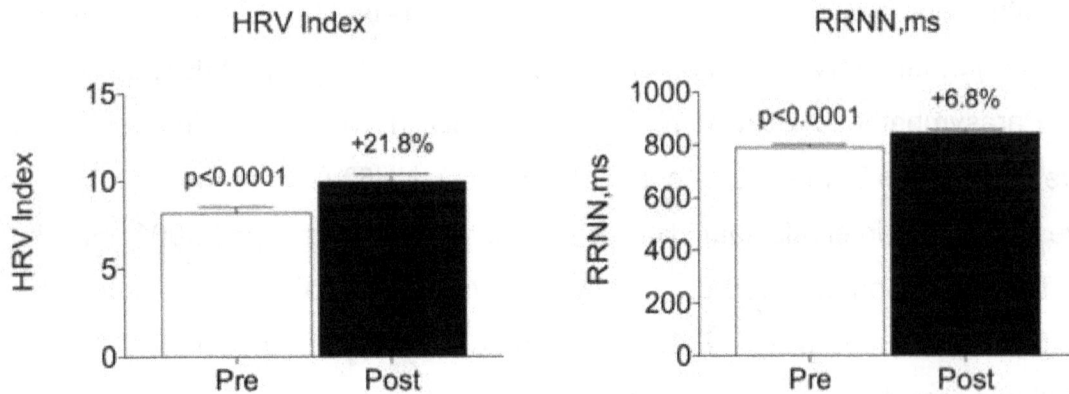

Figure 1: Effects of ABE on Heart Rate Variability Index and RRNN (RR normal-to-normal intervals; a marker of overall HRV activity). Paired T-Test 95% with a confidence interval (Graphpad Prism software, USA).

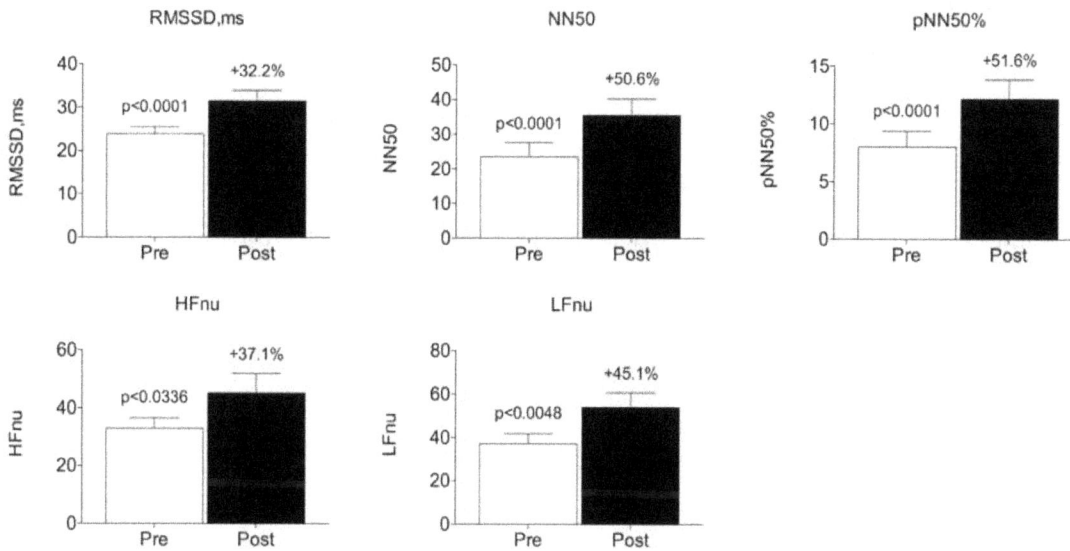

Figure 2: Effects of ABE on Parasympathetic activity markers. RMSSD (Root Mean Square of the Successive RR interval Differences; a marker of Parasympathetic activity); NN50 (The number of pairs of successive NN (R-R) intervals that differ by more than 50 ms; a marker of Parasympathetic activity); pNN50% (The proportion of NN50 divided by the total number of NN (R-R) intervals; a marker of Parasympathetic activity); HFnu (High Frequency Band: index of modulation of the parasympathetic branch of the autonomic nervous system); LFnu: (Low Frequency Band: general indicator of aggregate modulation of both the sympathetic and parasympathetic branches of the Autonomic Nervous System). Paired T-Test 95% with a confidence interval (Graphpad Prism software, USA).

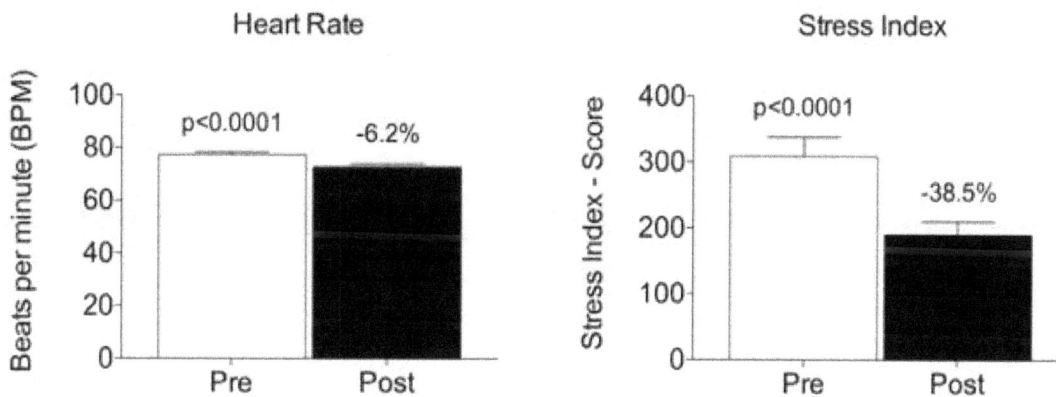

Figure 3: Effects of ABE on Heart Rate, Stress Index. Paired T-Test 95% with a confidence interval (Graphpad Prism software, USA).

5.1.7. Study #7. Presented at the Evidence based Non-invasive Therapies Conference in New Delhi, India, NOV 2019 (EBNITCON-2019).

Title
Effect of Audio-Visual Brain Entrainment on the Chakra system through data pulse analysis.

Author
Patrick K. Porter[1,2], Michael Porter[1], Francisco J Cidral-Filho[1]

1. Laboratory of Experimental Neurosciences. University of Southern Santa Catarina, SC, Brazil.
2. Postgraduate Program in Integrative Medicine. Quantum University. Honolulu, HI, USA.

Background
Audio Visual Brainwave entrainment (ABWE) is the synchronization of brainwaves with entraining stimuli, i.e., rhythmic visual (flickering lights) and auditory (Isochronic tones, and/or Binaural beats), that elicit synchronization of neural oscillations. The chakra system refers to the various focal points in the subtle body used in a variety of ancient meditation practices and integrative energy-based therapies.

Objective
The objective of this study was to investigate the effect of Audio-Visual Brain Entrainment (ABWE) on the Chakra system through data pulse analysis.

Methods
100 adult volunteers (50 males and 50 females) with no hearing disabilities were subjected to a single 20-minute ABE session with the BrainTap headset (New Bern - NC - USA). ABE consisted of Binaural beats at 18 to 0.5 HZ, Isochronic Tones at 18 to 0.5

HZ and visual Entrainment of light-emitting diode lights (470 nanometers - nm) flickering at 18 to 0.5 HZ. Data pulse analysis (NeuralChek, New Bern, NC, USA) was assessed at baseline and after ABE session.

Results

ABE significantly increased all chakras energy level in comparison to baseline evaluations, as assessed by Data Pulse Analysis. Root Chakra (Muladhara; $p<0.001$, 32.6%); Sacral Chakra (Svadhisthana; $p<0.001$, 36%); Solar Plexus Chakra (Manipura; $p<0.001$, 35.1%); Heart Chakra (Anahata; $p<0.001$, 44.5%); Throat Chakra (Vissudha; $p<0.001$, 28.9%); Third eye Chakra (Ajna; $p<0.001$, 40.7%); Crown Chakra (Sahasrara; $p<0.001$, 36%).

Conclusion

Audio-Visual Brain Entrainment with the BrainTap Headset significantly increased all chakra energy levels.

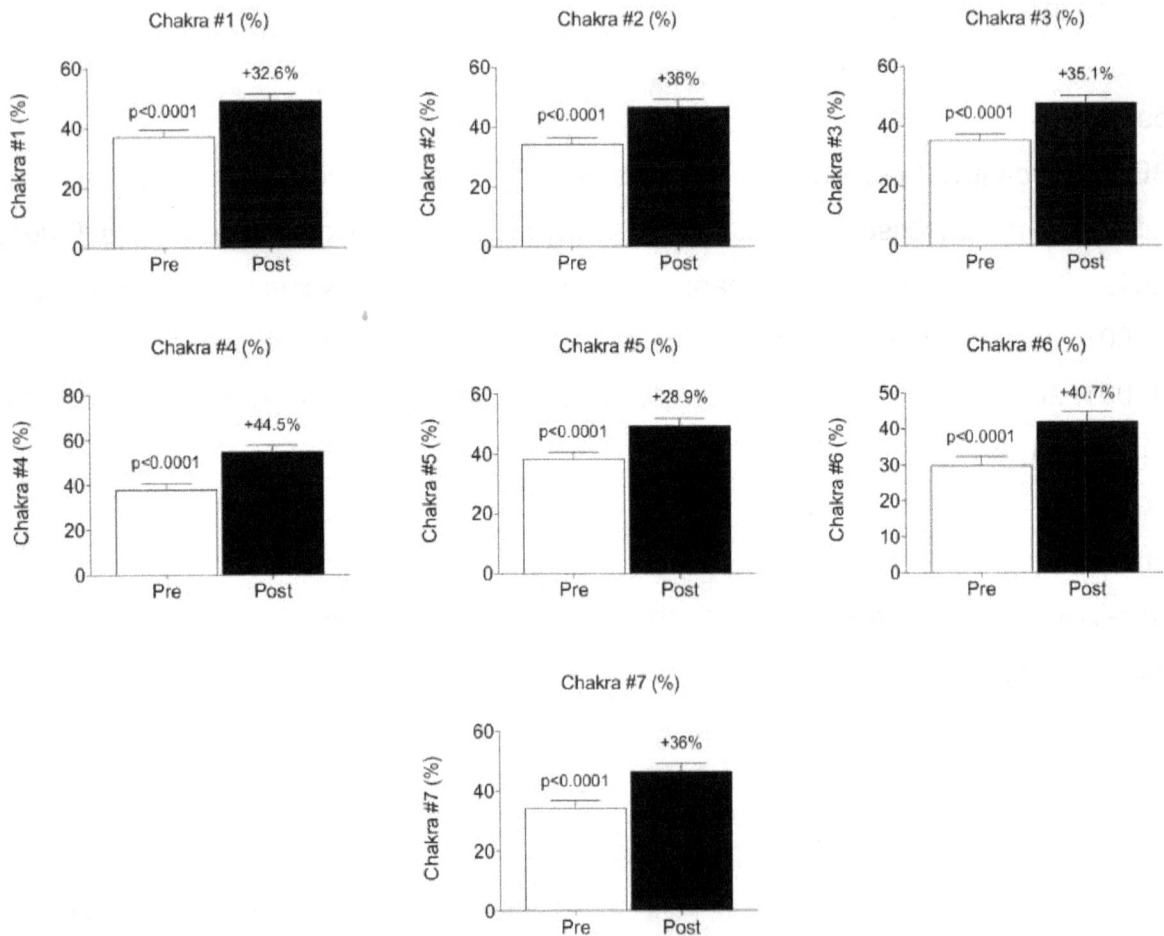

Figure 1 - The effect of Audio-Visual Brain Entrainment on the Chakra system through data pulse analysis. Paired T-Test 95% with a confidence interval (Graphpad Prism software, v.8, La Jolla, CA, USA).

5.2. PhD thesis

5.2.1. Study #8. PhD Thesis in the 2022 postgraduate Program in Integrative Medicine at the Quantum University, Honolulu, HI, USA.

Title

Effects of the Ready 4 Rapid Results H.E.A.L.T.H.Y. H.A.B.I.T.S. 13-week program, either alone or in combination with Braintap Brainwave Entrainment (BWE), on Weight Loss; Quality of Sleep, Mood, Anxiety, and Stress.

Authors

Kim White[1], Cidral-Filho, F.J.[2]; Porter, P.[1]

1. Postgraduate Program in Integrative Medicine. Quantum University. Honolulu, HI, USA.
2. Laboratory of Experimental Neurosciences. University of Southern Santa Catarina, SC, Brazil.

Objective

To evaluate the effects of the Ready 4 Rapid Results H.E.A.L.T.H.Y. H.A.B.I.T.S. 13-week program, either alone or in combination with Braintap Brainwave Entrainment (BWE), on Weight Loss; Quality of Sleep, Mood, Anxiety & Stress.

Background

The Ready 4 Rapid Results H.E.A.L.T.H.Y. H.A.B.I.T.S. 13-week program includes guidance for eating, moving, and thinking differently to reduce body weight and lead a healthier lifestyle. This guidance is based upon over 20 years of practice, research, and implementation of a healthy system.

Methods

Participants were screened and asked to sign this Consent Form. Participants then took the baseline evaluations: weight measurements as well as questionnaires (Pittsburgh Quality of Sleep Index - PQSI, Perceived Stress Scale - PSS, Generalized Anxiety Disorder 7 - GAD7, Profile of Mood States - POMS), and were randomly assigned to the intervention groups (GROUP HH or HH+BWE) with a computer-based random number generator (www.randomizer.org). Group HH participants underwent the Ready4Rapid program for 13 weeks, Group HH+BWE did so I combination with daily BWE sessions with the Braintap APP. All participants were re-evaluated after 3 and 6 weeks, i.e., midway and at the end of the intervention. Participants participated in the Ready 4 Rapid Results program by watching weekly videos, completing exercises and paperwork. They had weekly 1-hour meetings and a 15-minute Coaching Call or Zoom. BWE Group underwent daily 20-minute Brainwave Entrainment sessions.

Results

17 participants were initially enrolled, but only 9 completed the program and all 3 evaluations, 4 in HH group and 5 in HH+BWE group. Both groups presented weight reduction (from 3.4 To 5.6 pounds at the end of the experiment) with no statistically significant differences between groups (Figure 1). Although Quality of Sleep was not affected, both groups presented positively better scores in the POMS, PSS and GAD-7 questionnaires in comparison to baseline, although statistically significant results were only present in the POMS and the GAD-7 questionnaire and only for the HH+BWE group (Figure 2). Lastly, both interventions positively influenced Mood, with statistically significant results in comparison to baseline in the Tension and POMS negatives subscales, as well as on the overall score in the BWE group (Figure 3).

Conclusion

The Ready 4 Rapid Results H.E.A.L.T.H.Y. H.A.B.I.T.S. 13-week program did not influence quality of sleep, but positively affected Weight Loss, Mood, Anxiety, Stress. As statistically significant results in comparison to the baseline evaluations were only obtained in the HH+BWE group, data suggests that Braintap Brainwave Entrainment potentiated the effects of the interventions. Taken together, these data suggest that Braintap Brainwave Entrainment is an effective adjuvant therapy for weight loss and mood management programs.

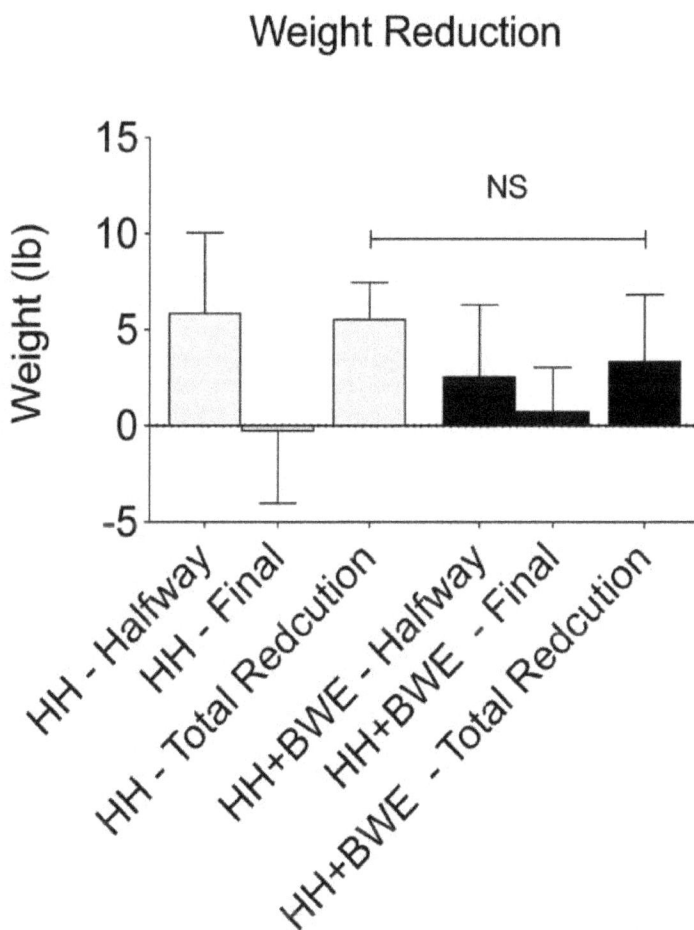

Figure 1 - Effects of the Ready 4 Rapid Results H.E.A.L.T.H.Y. H.A.B.I.T.S. 13-week program, either alone (HH) or in combination with Braintap Brainwave Entrainment (HH+BWE), on Weight Reduction. NS = Not statistically significant (Unpaired T-Test with a 95% confidence interval - Graphpad Prism software, USA).

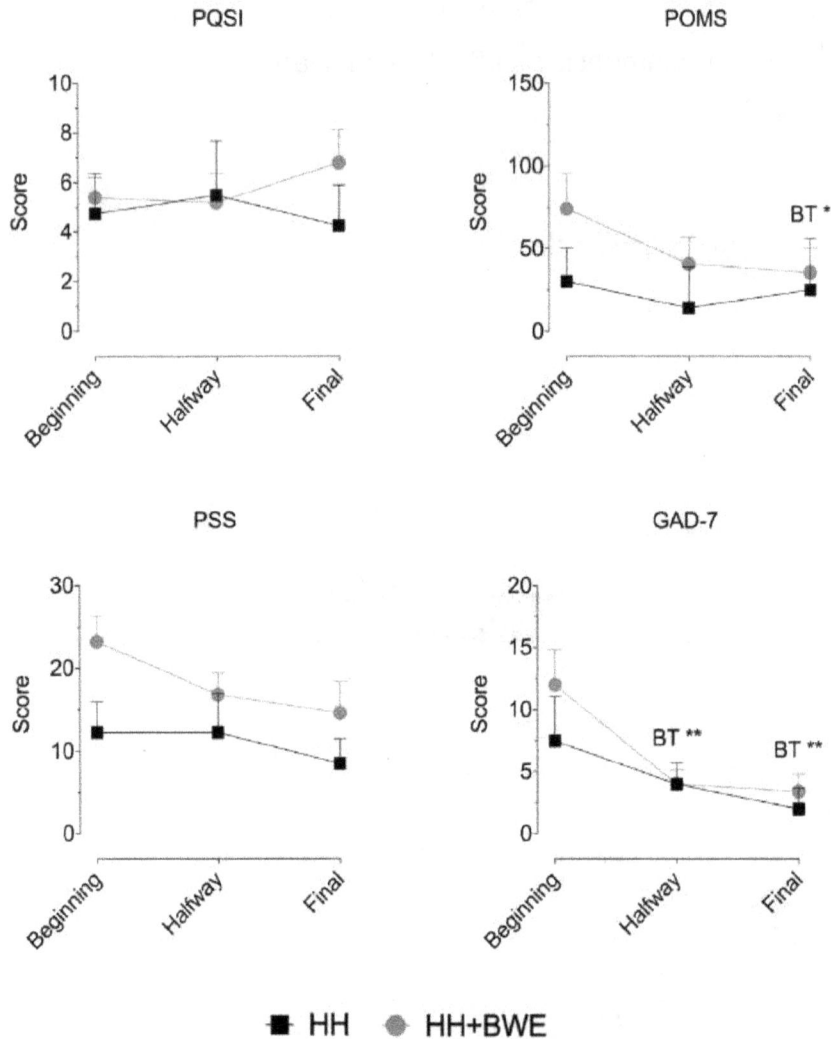

Figure 2 - Effects of the Ready 4 Rapid Results H.E.A.L.T.H.Y. H.A.B.I.T.S. 13-week program, either alone (HH) or in combination with Braintap Brainwave Entrainment (HH+BWE), on Quality of Sleep (PQSI), Mood (POMS), Anxiety (GAS-7) & Stress (PSS). NS = Not statistically significant, **$p < 0.01$ (Two-way ANOVA repeated measures followed by Bonferroni Post-hoc Test - Graphpad Prism software, USA).

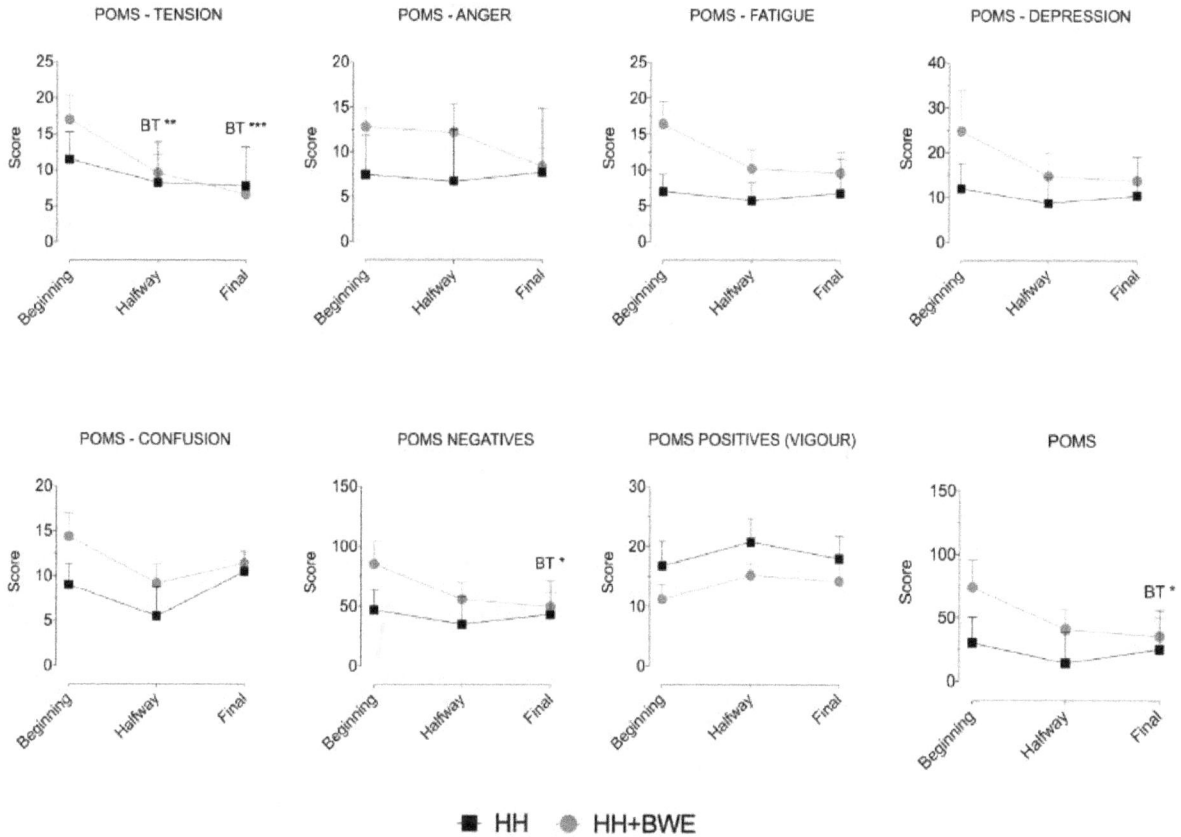

Figure 3 - Effects of the Ready 4 Rapid Results H.E.A.L.T.H.Y. H.A.B.I.T.S. 13-week program, either alone (HH) or in combination with Braintap Brainwave Entrainment (HH+BWE), on Mood (POMS subscales). NS = Not statistically significant, *p<0.05, **p<0.01, ***p<0.001 (Two-way ANOVA repeated measures followed by Bonferroni Post-hoc Test - Graphpad Prism software, USA).

5.2.2. Study #9. PhD Thesis in the 2021 postgraduate Program in Integrative Medicine at the Quantum University, Honolulu, HI, USA.

Title

Effect of audiovisual Brainwave Entrainment on Weight Reduction, Stress and Heart Rate variability.

Authors

Jody Dowd [1], Cidral-Filho, F.J.[2]; Porter, P.[1]

1. Postgraduate Program in Integrative Medicine. Quantum University. Honolulu, HI, USA.
2. Laboratory of Experimental Neurosciences. University of Southern Santa Catarina, SC, Brazil.

Objective

To evaluate the effect of audiovisual brainwave Entrainment (BWE) with the BrainTap headset on weight loss, stress, and heart rate variability.

Methods

Sample size consisted of 12 participants (three men and nine women, ages of 29 and 63, BMI of at least 30, who wanted to lose at least 15 pounds. Baseline assessments consisted of body weight (Health O Meter, USA), stress and heart rate variability (through the Neuralchek device, New Bern, USA). Participants were then asked to listen to two BWE sessions from the Braintap Application of their choice each day (one in the morning - in the Motivation category) and one in the evening (in the Relaxation category) with two of them being Weight Loss category sessions each week.

Results

12 participants were initially enrolled, but only 8 completed the program and the evaluations. A weight reduction of 2.125 pounds was recorded at the end of the program ($p=0.0243$ - Figure 1), and stress index was also reduced (24.1%, although stress index data was not statistically significant $p=0.2013$ - Figure 2). Additionally, although not statistically significance was obtained, assessments also indicated increased HRV, increased parasympathetic activity and increased balance between sympathetic and parasympathetic (Figure 2), as decrease in the LF/HF ratio indicates vagal activation, with results closer to 1 (one) reflecting better sympathovagal balance.

Conclusion

Audiovisual Brainwave Entrainment positively affected Weight Reduction. Results also indicate a positive effect on stress and Heart rate variability (with increased HRV, increased parasympathetic activity and increased sympathovagal balance), although data was not statistically significant, we argue that a larger size study is awarded.

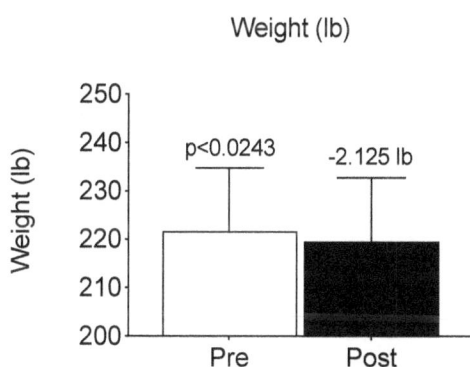

Figure 1 - Effect of audiovisual Brainwave Entrainment on Weight Reduction. Paired T-Test with a 95% confidence interval - Graphpad Prism software, USA.

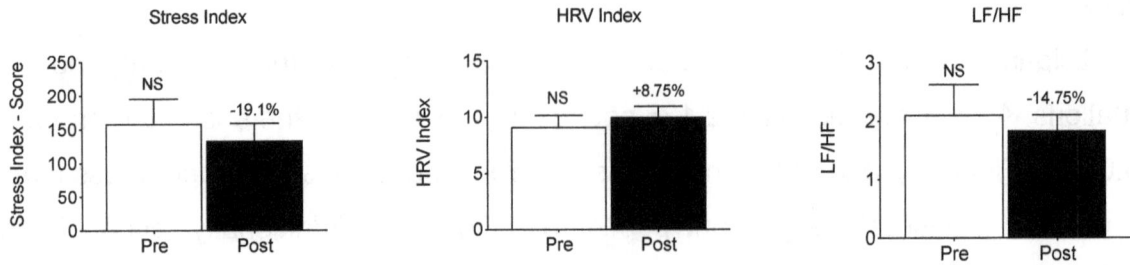

Figure 2 - Effect of audiovisual Brainwave Entrainment on Stress, Heart Rate Variability (HRV) and Low Frequency (LF) to High Frequency (HF) ratio. NS = Not statistically significant (Paired T-Test with a 95% confidence interval - Graphpad Prism software, USA).

5.3 Independent studies

5.3.1. Study #10. Internal study conducted with BioStrap & BrainTap team members. Conducted Online in 2021.

Title

Effect of Audio-Visual Brain Entrainment on Stress, Mood and Quality of Sleep: a trial with BioStrap & BrainTap team members.

Authors

Kevin Longoria[1]; Erin Miller[2]; Francisco Cidral[2,3]

1. BioStrap LLC, Los Angeles CA
2. Braintap Technologies, New Bern NC - USA.
3. Experimental Neuroscience Laboratory (LaNEx), University of Southern Santa Catarina (UNISUL), Brazil.

Objective

The study Objective was to investigate the effects of the Audio-Visual Brain Entrainment (ABE) on Stress, Mood and Quality of Sleep of BioStrap & BrainTap team members.

Methods

Sample size consisted of 32 volunteers who were not making use of analgesics, anti-inflammatories or sleep aids at least seven (7) days prior to, as well as during the study, and who had no hearing disabilities. Study was conducted over the course of 5 weeks. During weeks 1 and 2 (From May 5th to 18th): Baseline Evaluation Phase. Participants were asked NOT to undergo BWE sessions. During weeks 3, 4 and 5 (From May 19th to June 9th): Intervention phase. Participants were asked to undergo two (2) Braintap sessions a day. Assessments consisted of (1) online questionnaires and (2) "Sleep

Tracking with the Biostrap device". Online questionnaire consisted of five (5) parts: Part 1: Questions on the use of Braintap and overall health and wellness questions; Part 2: Pittsburgh Quality of Sleep Index: to access Quality of Sleep - as a counterpoint to BioStrap. Part 3: Perceived Stress Scale: to measure the perception of stress. Part 4: The Brief Resilience Scale: to assess the ability to bounce back or recover from stress. Part 5: Profile of Mood States: a widespread instrument which measures mood. The questionnaires were conducted on the following dates: On May 5th: Baseline Questionnaires; On May 19th: Beginning of Intervention Questionnaires; On June 9th: End of Study Questionnaires. (2) Sleep Tracking with the Biostrap device: The participants were asked to wear the BioStrap Band during the two phases of the study (Baseline and Intervention). ABE sessions were delivered with the BrainTap App and/or a BrainTap headset (New Bern - NC - USA) in 20 to 30-minute sessions twice (2x) a day during the intervention phase (from May 19th to June 9th). The sessions entailed background music, guided meditation, as well as audio or audiovisual brainwave entrainment through binaural beats, isochronic tones and, in the case of the use of the headset, photic stimulation. Results indicate that Audio-Visual Brain Entrainment (ABE):

- Significantly decreased Stress and increased Quality of Sleep, Perceived stress and Mood (as assessed through validated research questionnaires - Figures 1, 2 and 3) but did not affect Resilience (Brief Resilience Scale - Figure 2B);

- Significantly increased quality of sleep, mood, energy levels; decreased the feeling of being nervous and stressed, annoyed or irritable; and increased the feeling of being "on top of things" and productive (as assessed through self-reported 10-point Likert scale - Figure 4);

- In regards to the data assessed with the BioStrap Bands, although results were trending to on a positive direction, data were not statistically significant [resting heart rate, resting Heart rate variability (HRV), peripheral capillary oxygen saturation (SpO2), respiratory rate, arterial elasticity, peripheral elasticity, arterial age, sleep duration, seep efficiency (%), deep sleep (in minutes), light sleep (in minutes), total time Awake (in minutes), sleep awakenings (number of events), sleep Score (0-100 scale), recovery Score (0-100 scale) - Figures 5 through 8].

In relation to adherence to Braintapping during the intervention phase of study, "end of the study questionnaire" yielded the results (Figure 9):

- 52.4% of the participants consistently BrainTapped twice (2x) a day during intervention phase; 47.6% did not.
- 9.5% of the participants reported undergoing zero (0) BrainTap sessions a day; 33.3%, one session; and 57.1%, two sessions a day. No participants underwent three sessions a day.
- 19% of the participants generally used only the App; 81% generally the APP + Headset; and 4.8% of the participants did not generally BrainTap.

Conclusion

Overall results indicate that ABE significantly decreased Stress, increased Quality of Sleep, Mood and energy levels. Actigraphy data collected with the BioStrap Bands, although not statistically significant, indicated improvement in all parameters analyzed.

Limitations of this trial are (1) inconsistent participation during the intervention phase, the small sample size, and the fact that the study was not placebo-controlled.

A randomized blinded placebo-controlled trial with a lager sample size study is awarded to confirm the effects of ABE.

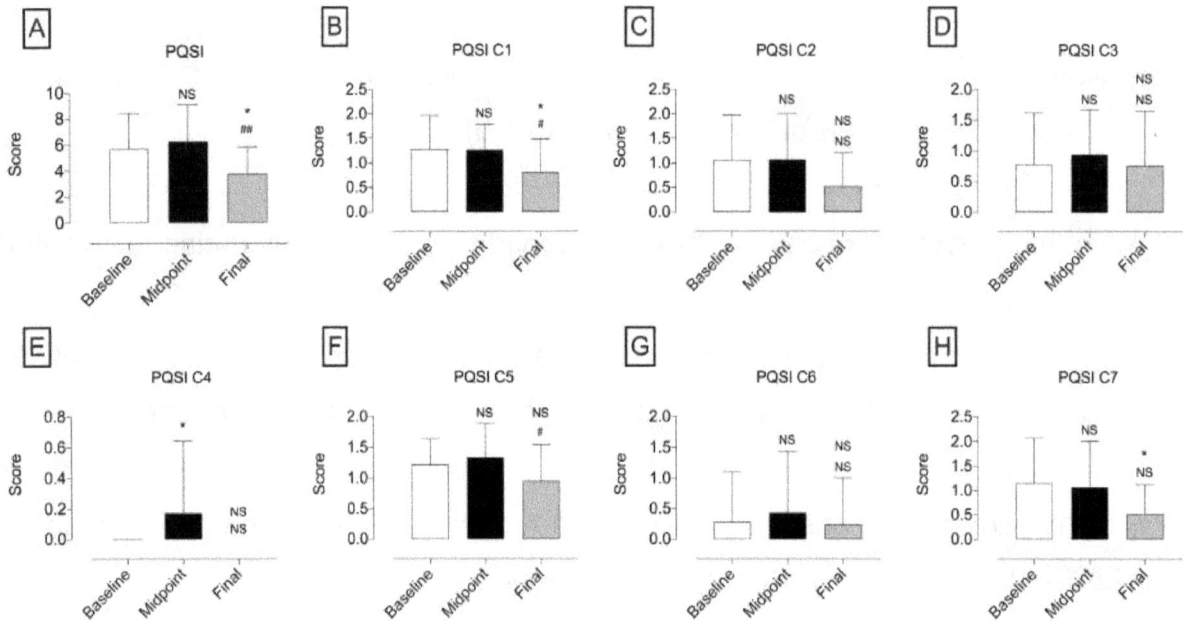

Figure 1. Pittsburgh Quality of Sleep Index (PQSI). Global PSQI Score (Panel A); Component 1 (C1 - Panel B): Subjective sleep quality; Component 2 (C2 - Panel C): Sleep latency; Component 3 (C3 - Panel D): Sleep duration; Component 4 (C4 - Panel E): Sleep efficiency; Component 5 (C5 - Panel F): Sleep disturbance; Component 6 (C6 - Panel G): Use of sleep medication; Component 7 (C7 - Panel H): Daytime dysfunction. NS: Not statistically significant. *$p < 0.05$ when compared to baseline evaluation, #$p < 0.05$ when compared to midpoint Evaluation. Ordinary One-Way Anova followed by Tukey's multiple comparisons test or Kruskal-Wallis test followed by Dunn's multiple comparisons test, where applicable (prism graphpad 8, La Jola USA).

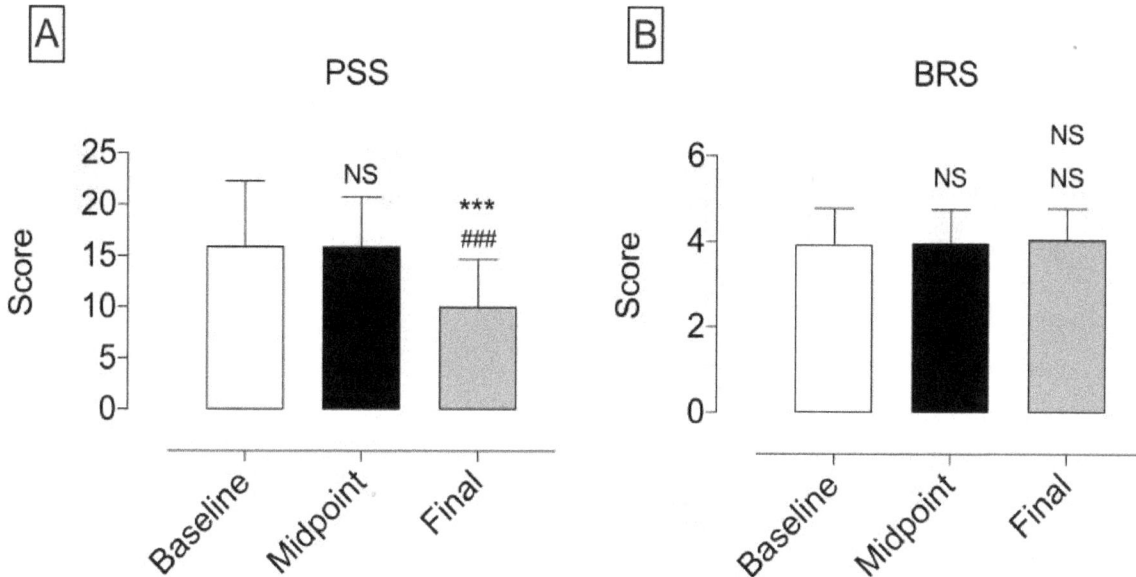

Figure 2. Perceived Stress Scale (Panel A); The Brief Resilience Scale (Panel B). NS: Not statistically significant. ***p<0.001 when compared to baseline evaluation, ###p<0.001 when compared to midpoint Evaluation Ordinary One-Way Anova followed by Tukey's multiple comparisons test (prism graphpad 8, La Jola USA).

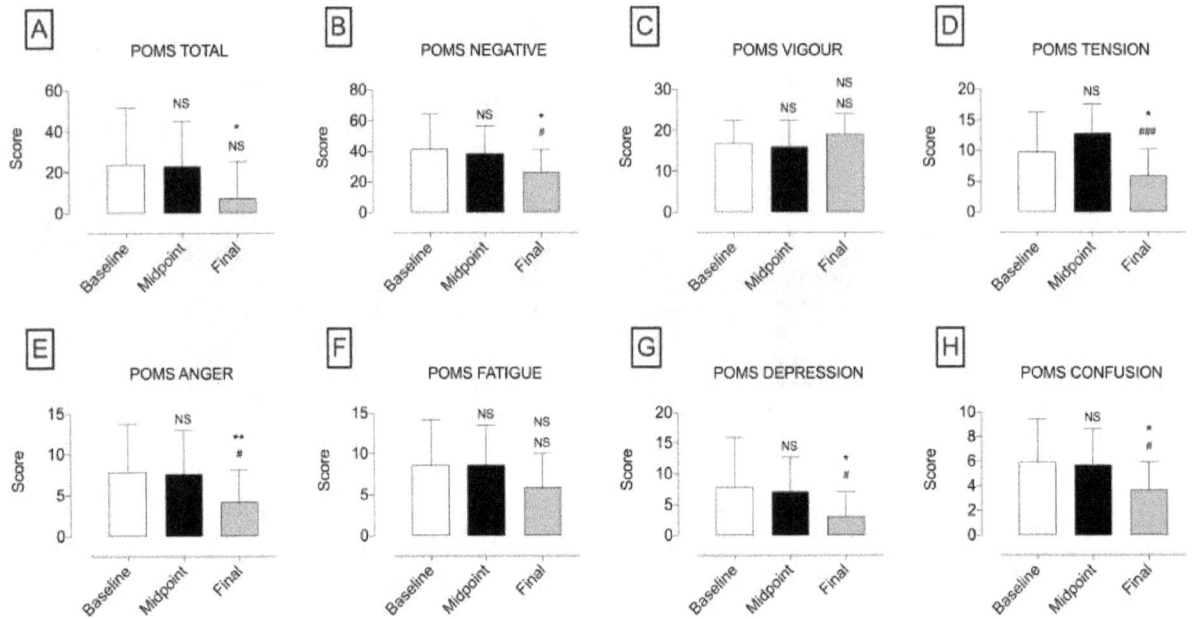

Figure 3. Profile of Mood States (POMS). Total score (Panel A); POMS Negative Aspects (Panel B); Vigor score (Panel C); Tension score (Panel D); Anger score (Panel E); Fatigue score (Panel F); Depression score (Panel G); Confusion score (Panel H). NS: Not statistically significant. *$p<0.05$, **$p<0.01$ when compared to baseline evaluation, #$p<0.05$, ###$p<0.001$ when compared to midpoint Evaluation. Ordinary One-Way Anova followed by Tukey's multiple comparisons test or Kruskal-Wallis test followed by Dunn's multiple comparisons test, where applicable (prism graphpad 8, La Jola USA).

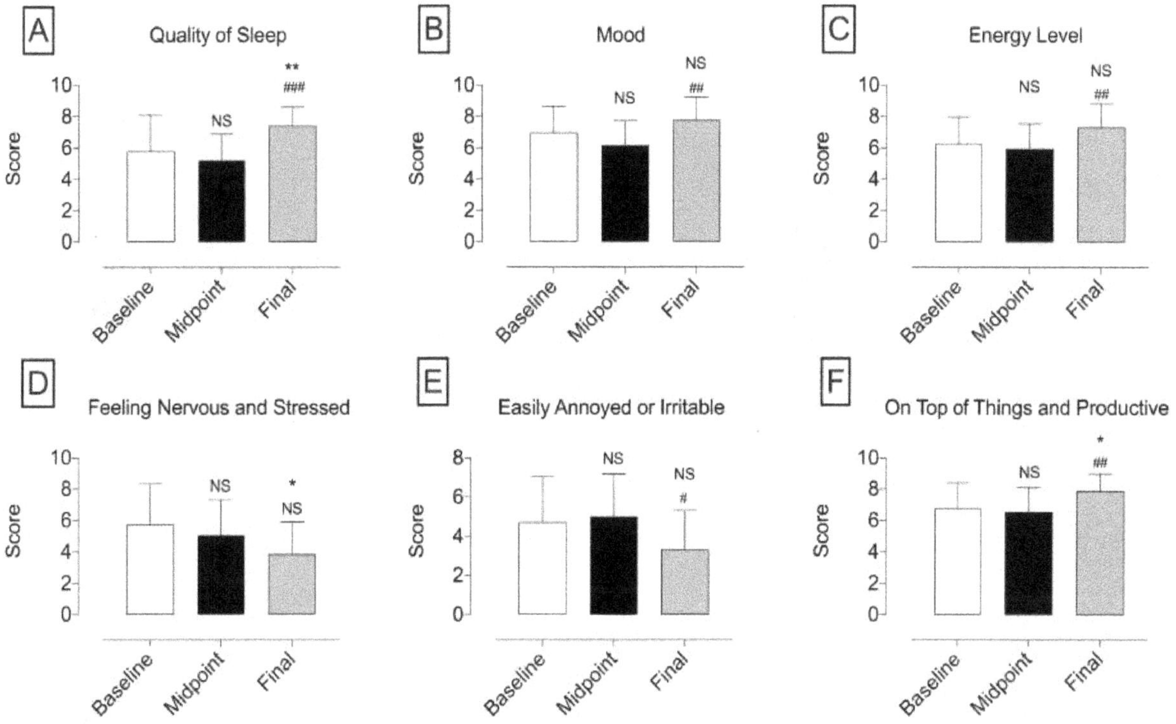

Figure 4. Self-reported 10-point Likert scale. Quality of sleep (Panel A); Mood (Panel B); Energy levels (Panel C); Feeling of being nervous and stressed (Panel D); Feeling of being annoyed or irritable (Panel E); Feeling of being "on top of things" and productive (Panel F). NS: Not statistically significant. *p<0.05, **p<0.01 when compared to baseline evaluation, ##p<0.01, ###p<0.001 when compared to midpoint Evaluation. Ordinary One-Way Anova followed by Tukey's multiple comparisons test or Kruskal-Wallis test followed by Dunn's multiple comparisons test, where applicable (prism graphpad 8, La Jola USA).

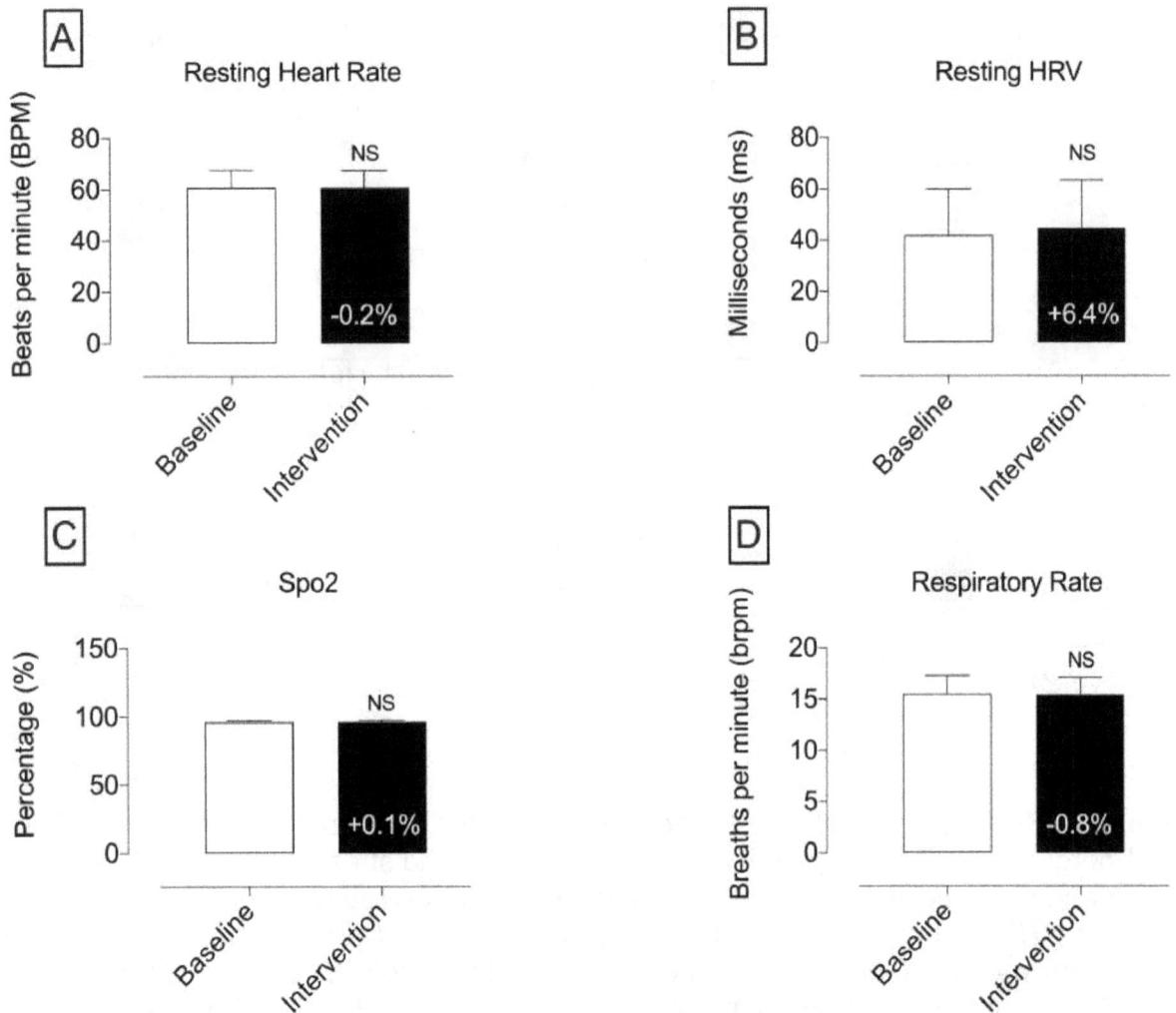

Figure 5. Biostrap data. Resting heart rate (Panel A); Resting Heart rate variability (HRV) (Panel B); Peripheral capillary oxygen saturation (SpO_2) (Panel C); Respiratory rate (Panel D). NS: Not statistically significant. Unpaired or paired t test or Wilcoxon matched-pairs signed rank test, where applicable (prism graphpad 8, La Jola USA).

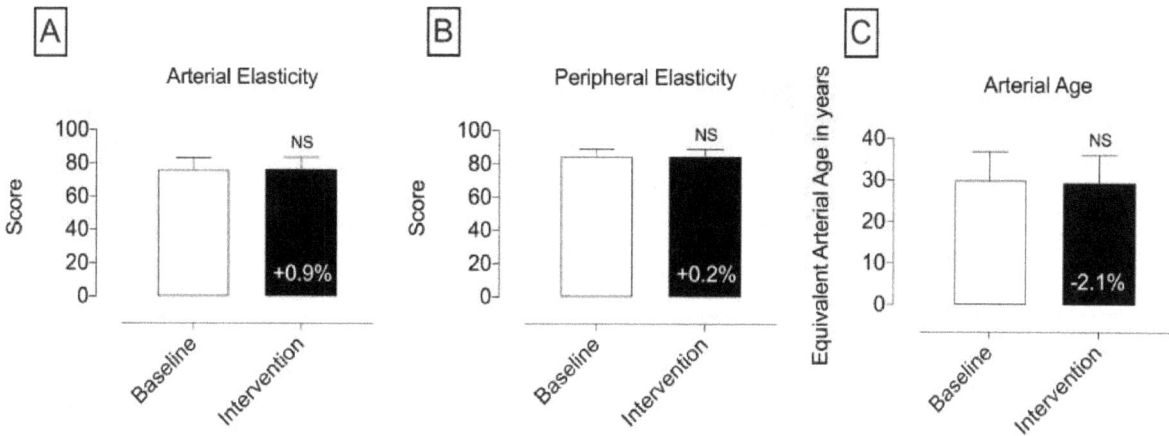

Figure 6. Biostrap data. Arterial elasticity (Panel A); Peripheral elasticity (Panel B); Arterial age (Panel C). NS: Not statistically significant. Unpaired or paired t test or Wilcoxon matched-pairs signed rank test, where applicable (prism graphpad 8, La Jola USA).

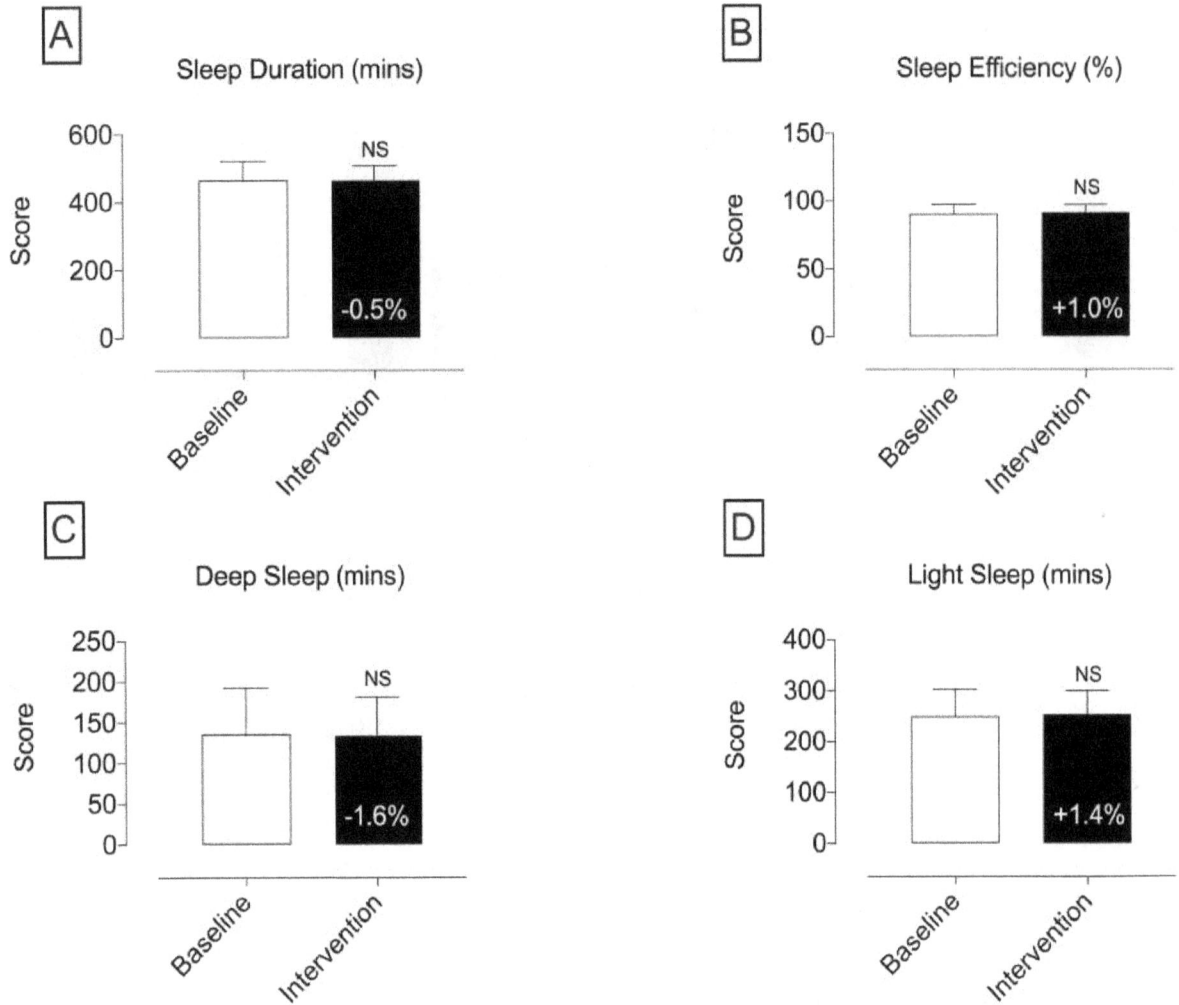

Figure 7. Biostrap data. Sleep duration (Panel A); Seep efficiency (%) (Panel B); Deep sleep (Panel C); Light sleep (Panel D). NS: Not statistically significant. Unpaired or paired t test or Wilcoxon matched-pairs signed rank test, where applicable (prism graphpad 8, La Jola USA).

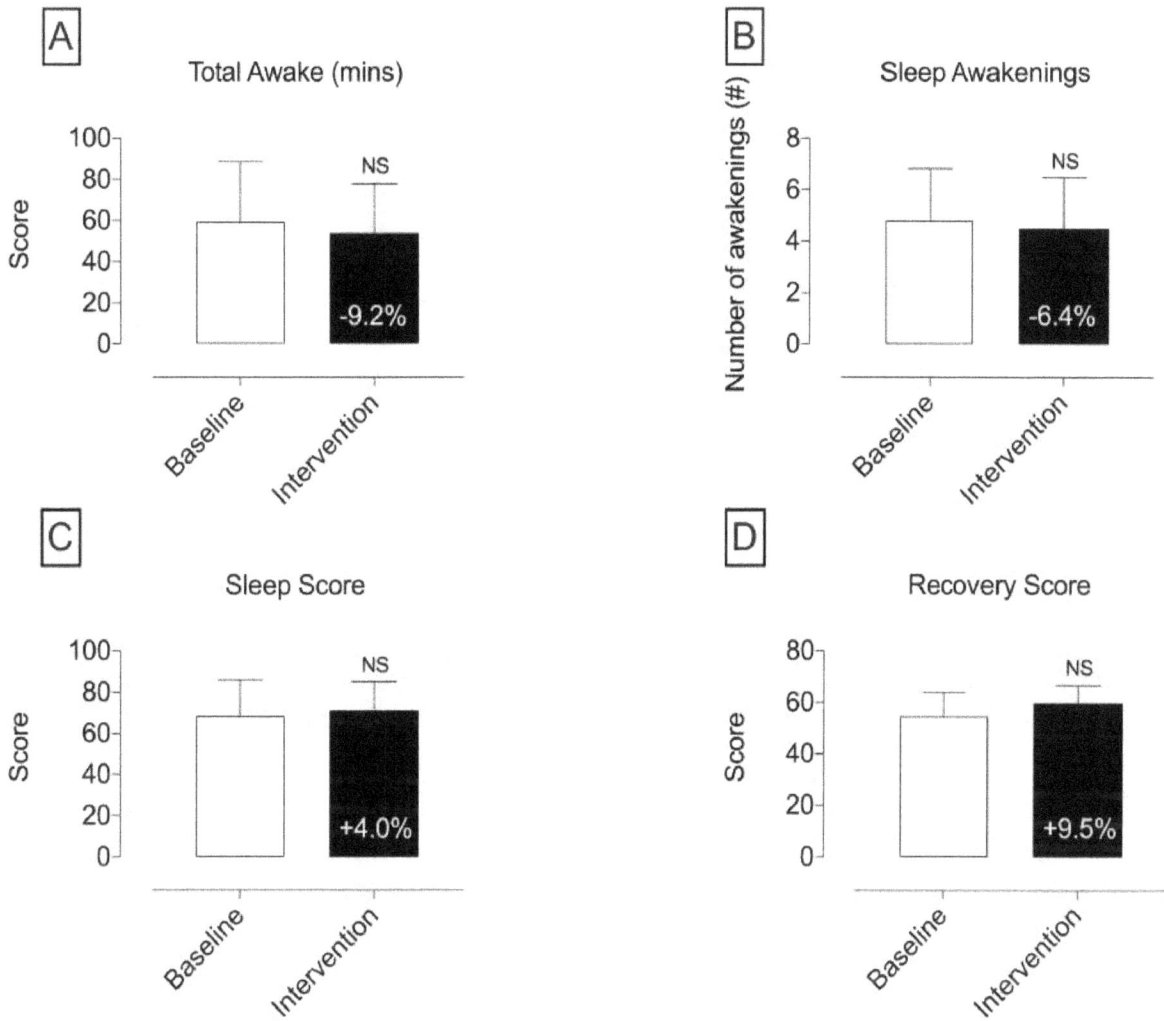

Figure 8. Biostrap data. Total time Awake (Panel A); Sleep awakenings (Panel B); Sleep Score (Panel C); Recovery Score (Panel D). NS: Not statistically significant. Unpaired or paired t test or Wilcoxon matched-pairs signed rank test, where applicable (prism graphpad 8, La Jola USA).

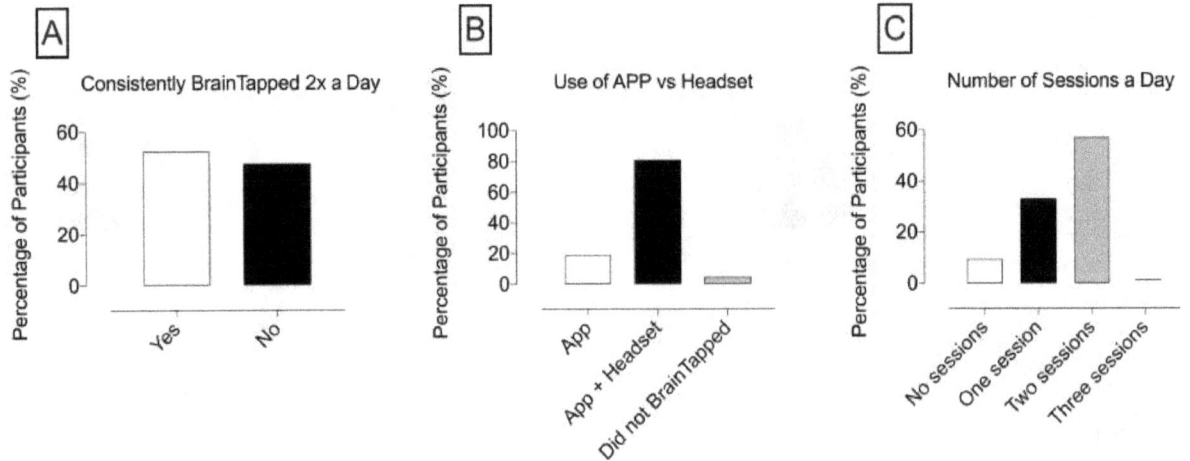

Figure 9. Adherence to Braintapping during the intervention phase of study. Consistently BrainTapped twice (2x) a day during intervention phase (Panel A); Use of App versus Headset (Panel B); Number of Sessions a day (Panel C).

5.3.2. Study #11. Study conducted by Dr. Arkfeld at the Gaylord High School in Gaylord, MI, United States. 2020-2021.

Title

Concussion Treatment Protocol Utilizing Brainwave Entrainment with the BrainTap headset & Compression Therapy with the NormaTec Pulse 2.0.

Authors

Arkfeld T.[1], Cidral-Filho, F.J.[2]; Porter, P.[1]

1. Postgraduate Program in Integrative Medicine. Quantum University. Honolulu, HI, USA.
2. Laboratory of Experimental Neuroscience (LANEX) - Health Sciences Post-Graduation Program - University of Southern Santa Catarina (UNISUL), Brazil.

Objective

Evaluate the effect of Brainwave Entrainment (BWE) with the BrainTap headset and compression therapy (CT) with the NormaTec Pulse 2.0 Legs device as adjuvant to the treatment of sports-related concussion in high school athletes from boys and girls soccer, boys and girls basketball, girls softball, football, and cheerleaders.

Methods

Control group patients (n=6) who sustained a sports-related concussion and were under care for concussion-related symptoms were treated with low force chiropractic manipulations, electrical muscle stimulation, and neuromuscular reeducation exercises using the oscillating technique for isometric stabilization tools. During the first 10 days of intervention patients were seen daily, then the frequency was reduced to 3 times per week until release from active care (which varied based on the individual patient's response to care). BWE+CT group (n=10) received same interventions as the Control group along with BWE with the BrainTap Headset in combination with CT with the NormaTec Pulse

2.0 Legs device. In the first 10 days of intervention BWE sessions consisted of Sensorimotor Rhythm (SMR) recordings, either 10 or 20 minutes in duration. From the 10th day onwards the "Stress Relief" series in the Braintap App were used. All BWE sessions were conducted in conjunction with CT with the NormaTec Pulse 2.0 Legs device. One year after the interventions ceased and the patients had been released from care, they were asked to complete a Post-Concussion Assessment on the lingering effects they were still experiencing.

Results

BWE+CT group reported less severe symptoms in all items, with a reduction from 30 to 90% in relation to Control group. Statistically significant differences between the groups were found in the following items: neck pain ($p < 0.05$), dizziness ($p < 0.05$), balance problems ($p < 0.01$), sensitivity to noise ($p < 0.05$), fatigue or low energy ($p < 0.01$), feeling more emotional ($p < 0.05$), and irritability ($p < 0.05$) (Figures 1-4).

Conclusion

The combination of Brainwave Entrainment (BWE) with the BrainTap headset and compression therapy (CT) with NormaTec Pulse 2.0 Legs device effectively reduced the long-lasting or lingering symptoms of sports-related concussion in high school athletes from boys and girls soccer, boys and girls basketball, girls softball, football, and cheerleaders in comparison to Control group interventions. Better results were seen more than a year after the interventions.

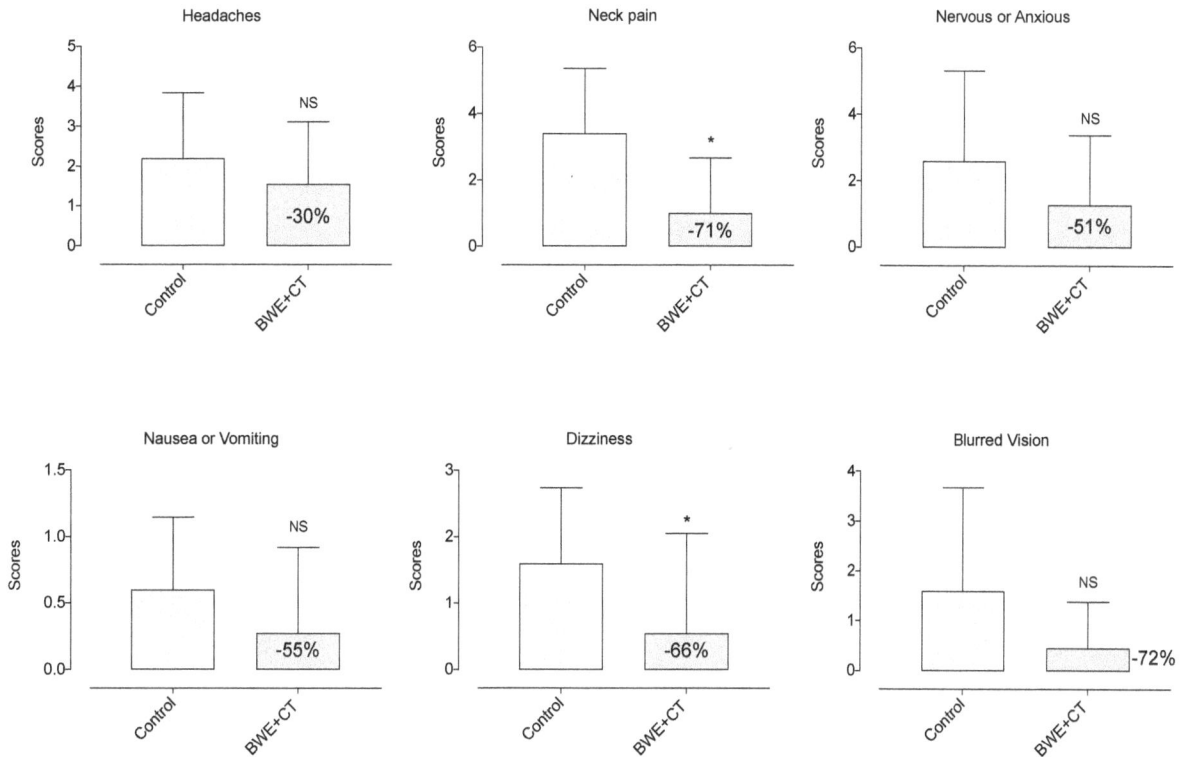

Figure 1 - The combination of Brainwave Entrainment (BWE) with the BrainTap headset and compression therapy (CT) with NormaTec Pulse 2.0 Legs device effectively reduced the long-lasting or lingering symptoms of sports-related concussion in comparison to Control group interventions. NS = Not statistically significant. *$p<0.05$, **$p<0.01$ (paired T-Test 95% with a confidence interval - Graphpad Prism software, USA).

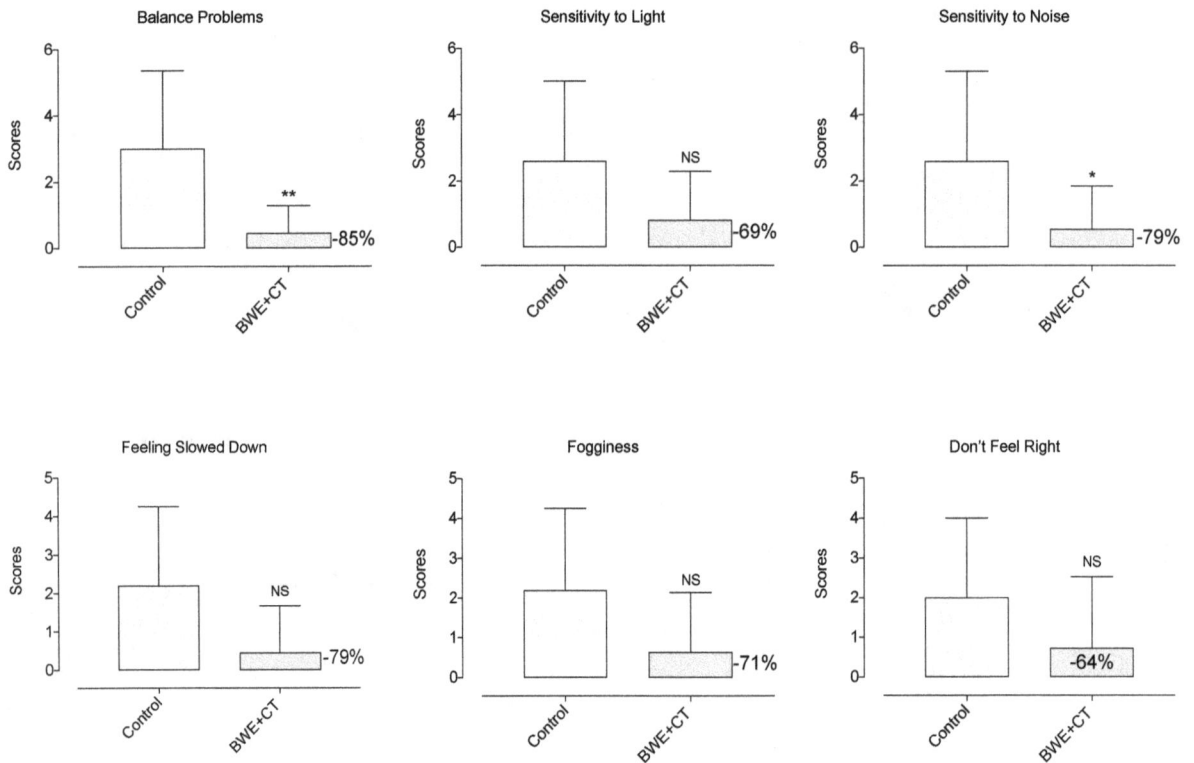

Figure 2 - The combination of Brainwave Entrainment (BWE) with the BrainTap headset and compression therapy (CT) with NormaTec Pulse 2.0 Legs device effectively reduced the long-lasting or lingering symptoms of sports-related concussion in comparison to Control group interventions. NS = Not statistically significant. *$p<0.05$, **$p<0.01$ (paired T-Test with a 95% confidence interval - Graphpad Prism software, USA).

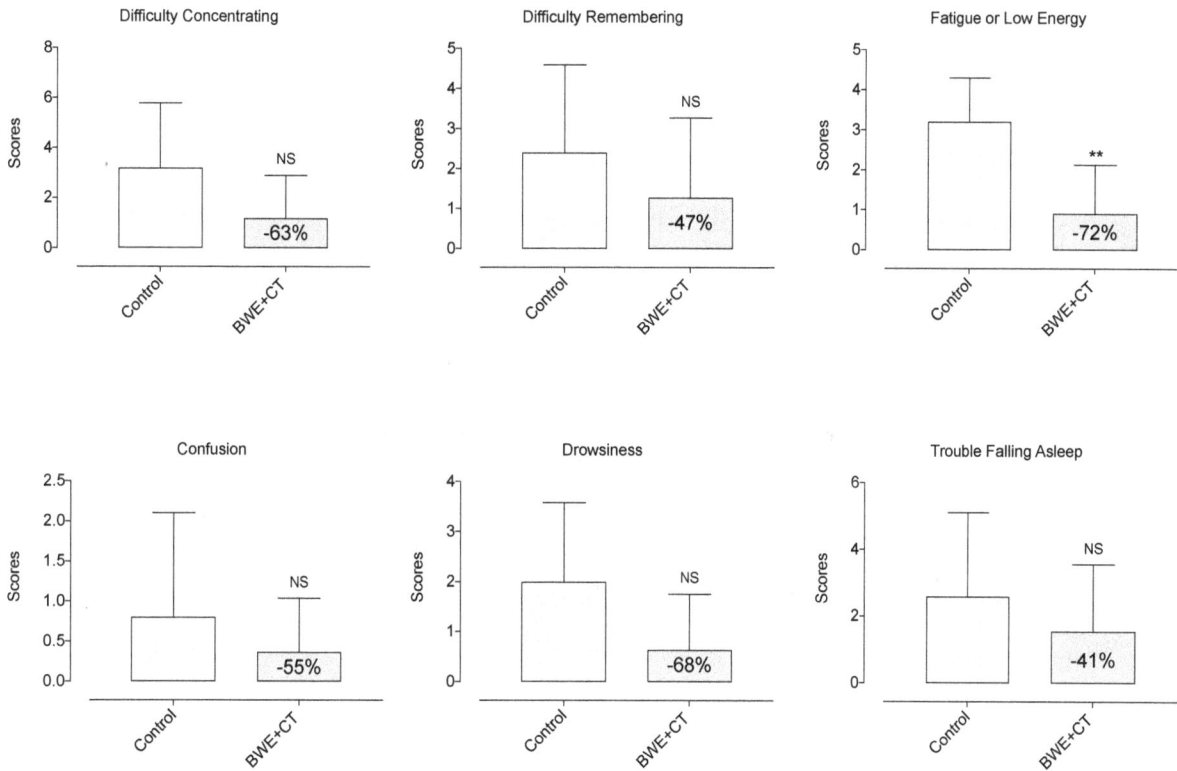

Figure 3 - The combination of Brainwave Entrainment (BWE) with the BrainTap headset and compression therapy (CT) with NormaTec Pulse 2.0 device effectively reduced the long-lasting or lingering symptoms of sports-related concussion in comparison to Control group interventions. NS = Not statistically significant. $*p<0.05$, $**p<0.01$ (paired T-Test with a 95% confidence interval - Graphpad Prism software, USA).

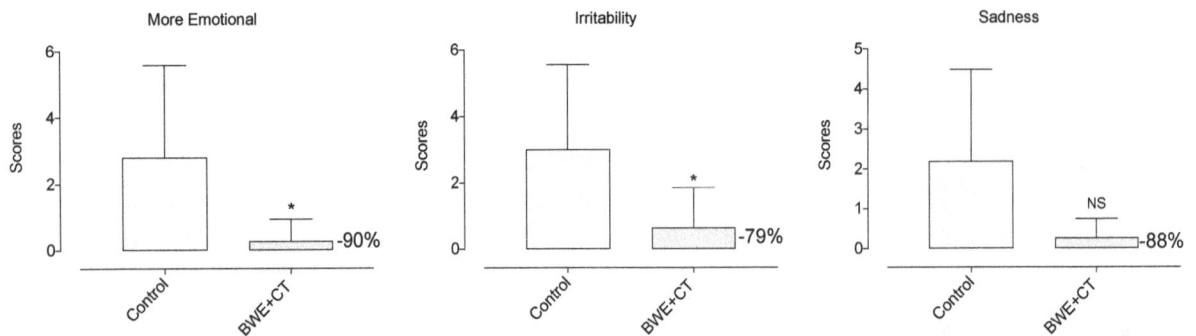

Figure 4 - The combination of Brainwave Entrainment (BWE) with the BrainTap headset and compression therapy (CT) with NormaTec Pulse 2.0 device effectively reduced the long-lasting or lingering symptoms of sports-related concussion in comparison to Control group interventions. NS = Not statistically significant. *$p<0.05$, **$p<0.01$ (paired T-Test with a 95% confidence interval - Graphpad Prism software, USA).

5.3.3. Study #12. Conducted with Julia Arndt (the Peak Performance Method creator - Conducted Online in 2020.

Title

The Effect of the Peak Performance Method (PPM) combined with Audio Brain Entrainment on Anxiety, Sleep, Stress and Work Productivity of Professionals.

Authors

Julia Arndt[1], Patrick K Porter[1], Francisco J Cidral-Filho[2]

1. Postgraduate Program in Integrative Medicine. Quantum University. Honolulu, HI.
2. Laboratory of Experimental Neurosciences. University of Southern Santa Catarina, Brazil.

Background

Developed by Julia Arndt, the Peak Performance Method (PPM) combines critical productivity, mindfulness and leadership tools with neuroscientific research on emotion regulation, habit-building and change management as well as coaching techniques to help people develop the next workplace superpower to thrive in today's high-pressure environments. Audio Brain Entertainment (ABWE) guides the mind from an awake, reactionary mind into an intuitive, creative state, then to a place where super-learning and healing can occur, with the outcome being a heightened state of consciousness with crystal clear focus. ABWE creates a symphony of brainwave activity, a feeling of calm focus for learning and productivity. Each session is designed with brainwave balance in mind. Unlike meditation programs, BrainTap's exclusive neuro-algorithms gently and naturally guide your brain through a broad range of brainwave patterns, instead of just the Alpha state. The result is a complete spectrum of brainwave activity.

Objective

The objective of this study was to investigate the effect of the Peak Performance Method (PPM) combined with Audio Brain Entrainment (ABWE) on Anxiety, General Health, Stress, Quality of Sleep, mindset and Work productivity of professionals.

Methods

Sample size consisted of 20 professionals of varying backgrounds (14 females and 6 males aged between 28 and 55). Professionals work in tech, consulting and telecommunication. 14 individuals are currently employed full-time, 5 individuals are self-employed and 1 not employed at the time. Group 1 and 2 learned the basics of PPM in 9 weekly pre-recorded 30-45-minute sessions, each session including a workbook with 3-5 journaling prompts for self-reflection and additional action items. Additionally, the participants were asked to complete a 5-minute reflection exercise at the end of each day to increase self-awareness and promote well-being. Furthermore, Group 2 deepened their learnings by adding 20-minute PPM-Braintap sessions 3 times a week for 9 weeks to influence their subconscious mind to make long-lasting changes in the following three areas: mindfulness, productivity and leadership.

The following questionnaires were applied at baseline and after 9 weeks to analyze the participants change in stress, sleep, mindset and productivity:

- Perceived Stress Scale (PSS);
- Pittsburgh Quality of Sleep Index (PQSI);
- Depression Scale (PQ-8);
- Mindset Scale by Carol Dweck;
- PPM Scale by Julia Arndt (not validated).

Results

PPM whether or not combined with ABWE positively affected all scores.

Results indicate positive effects of PPM on all scales evaluated. When PPM was combined with ABWE effects were more pronounced in most scales.

- PSS (33% reduction for PPM and 45% when combined with ABWE). In this scale a score of 0-13 indicates low stress levels; 14-26 - moderate stress and 27-40 - high perceived stress.

- PHQ-8 (18% reduction for PPM and 71% when combined with ABWE). Patient Health Questionnaire depression scale (PHQ-8) is established as a valid diagnostic and severity measure for depressive disorders. A score of 10 or greater is considered major depression, 20 or more is severe major depression. Statistically significant results were obtained in post-hoc analysis when comparing PPM+ABWE group with its baseline ($p<0.05$).

- PQSI (48% reduction for PPM and 51% when combined with ABWE). PQSI global score ranges from 0 to 21. Higher scores indicate worse sleep quality. Global sum of "5" or greater indicates a "poor" sleeper.

- Work Dimension (26% increase for PPM and 28% when combined with BrainTapping). The higher the score the better the outcome. Statistically significant results were obtained in post-hoc analysis when comparing PPM+ABWE group with its baseline ($p<0.05$).

- Mindset (41% increase for PPM and 19% when combined with ABWE). The higher the score the better the outcome.

- Beliefs and Values (10% increase for PPM and 3% when combined with ABWE). The higher the score the better the outcome.

Conclusion

Despite the reduced sample size (N=12 participants completed the study end-to-end) PPM positively affected scores related to anxiety, general health, stress, quality of sleep, as well as work productivity. Additionally, combining ABWE with PPM leads to more significant effects on most of the outcomes assessed in this study. Statistically significant results were obtained in post-hoc analysis when comparing PPM+ABWE group with its baseline ($p<0.05$) in two scales: PHQ-8 and Work Dimension assessments. A larger sample size study is necessary to statistically confirm the effects of PPM and the combination with ABWE.

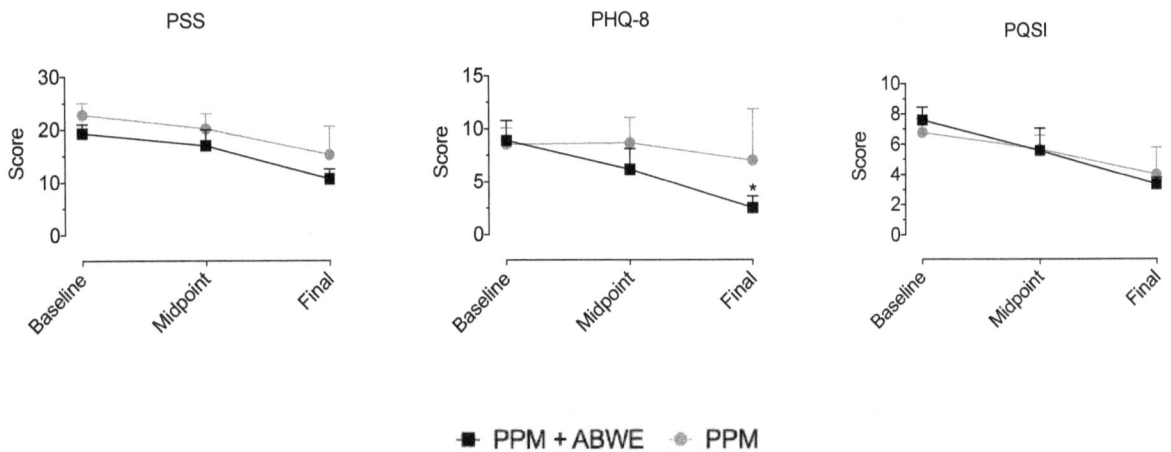

Figure 1: Effect of Peak Performance Method (PPM) and combination with Audio Brainwave Entrainment on Perceived Stress Scale (PSS), Patient Health Questionnaire (PHQ-8) and Pittsburgh Quality of Sleep Index (PQSI). *$p<0.05$ when comparing PPM+ABWE group with Baseline (Two-way ANOVA repeated Measures followed by Bonferroni Post-hoc analysis - prism Graphpad 9, La Jola, CA, USA).

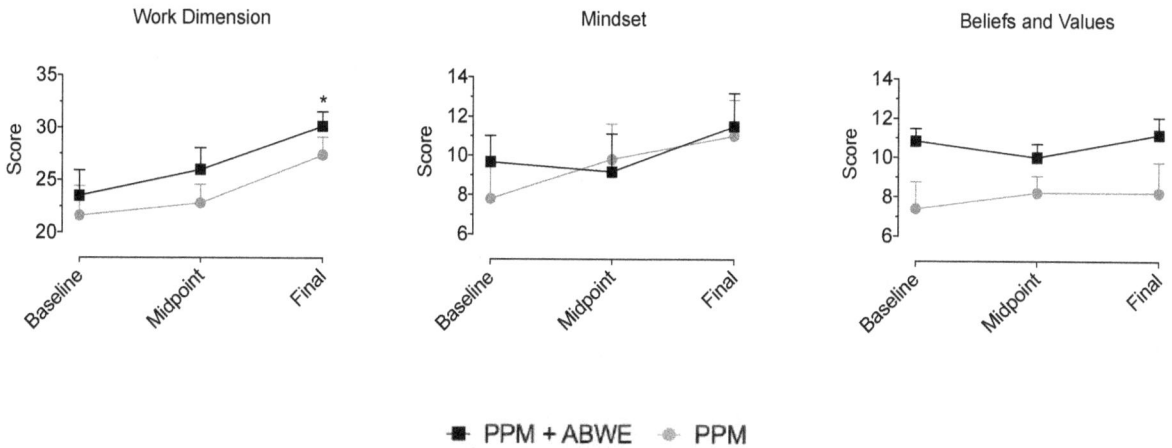

Figure 2: Effect of Peak Performance Method (PPM) and combination with ABWE on Work Dimension, Mindset and Beliefs and Values Assessment. *$p<0.05$ when comparing PPM+ABWE group with Baseline (Two-way ANOVA repeated Measures followed by Bonferroni Post-hoc analysis - prism Graphpad 9, La Jola, CA, USA).

6. References

1. Abeln V, Kleinert J, Strüder HK, Schneider S. Brainwave entrainment for better sleep and post-sleep state of young elite soccer players - a pilot study. Eur J Sport Sci. 2014;14(5):393-402. doi: 10.1080/17461391.2013.819384. Epub 2013 Jul 18. PubMed PMID: 23862643.

2. Adrian, E., & Matthews, B. The Berger rhythm: Potential changes from the occipital lobes of man. Brain, 57, 355–385, 1934.

3. Beauchene C, Abaid N, Moran R, Diana RA, Leonessa A. The effect of binaural beats on verbal working memory and cortical connectivity. J Neural Eng. 2017 Apr;14(2):026014. doi: 10.1088/1741-2552/aa5d67. Epub 2017 Feb 1. PMID: 28145275

4. Chaieb L, Wilpert EC, Hoppe C, Axmacher N, Fell J. The Impact of Monaural Beat Stimulation on Anxiety and Cognition. Front Hum Neurosci. 2017 May 15;11:251. doi: 10.3389/fnhum.2017.00251. eCollection 2017. PubMed PMID: 28555100; PubMed Central PMCID: PMC5430051.

5. Chaieb L, Wilpert EC, Reber TP, Fell J. Auditory beat stimulation and its effects on cognition and mood States. Front Psychiatry. 2015 May 12;6:70. doi: 10.3389/fpsyt 2015.00070. eCollection 2015. Review. PubMed PMID: 26029120; PubMed Central PMCID: PMC4428073.

6. Chatrian, E. G., Peterson, M. C., & Lazarte, J. A. (1960). Responses to clicks from the human brain: Some depth electrograph observation. Electroencephalography and Clinical Neurophysiology, 12, 479–489. doi:10.1016/0013-4694(60)90024-9.

7. Colzato LS, Barone H, Sellaro R, Hommel B. More attentional focusing through binaural beats: evidence from the global-local task. Psychol Res. 2017 Jan;81(1):271-277. doi: 10.1007/s00426-015-0727-0. Epub 2015 Nov 26. PubMed PMID: 26612201; PubMed Central PMCID: PMC5233742.

8. Derner M, Chaieb L, Surges R, Staresina BP, Fell J. Modulation of Item and Source Memory by Auditory Beat Stimulation: A Pilot Study With Intracranial EEG. Front Hum

Neurosci. 2018 Dec 11;12:500. doi: 10.3389/fnhum.2018.00500. eCollection 2018. PubMed PMID: 30618681; PubMed Central PMCID: PMC6297717.

9. Ecsy K, Brown CA, Jones AKP. Cortical nociceptive processes are reduced by visual alpha-band entrainment in the human brain. Eur J Pain. 2018 Mar;22(3):538-550. doi: 10.1002/ejp.1136. Epub 2017 Nov 14. PubMed PMID: 29139226.

10. Ecsy K, Jones AK, Brown CA. Alpha-range visual and auditory stimulation reduces the perception of pain. Eur J Pain. 2017 Mar;21(3):562-572. doi: 10.1002/ejp.960. Epub 2016 Nov 2. PubMed PMID: 27807916.

11. Ecsy Katharina. Analgesic effects of EEG alpha-wave entrainment on acute and chronic pain. Thesis submitted to The University of Manchester for the degree of Doctor of Philosophy in the Faculty of Medical and Human Sciences, 2014.

12. Garcia-Argibay M, Santed MA, Reales JM. Efficacy of binaural auditory beats in cognition, anxiety, and pain perception: a meta-analysis. Psychol Res. 2019 Mar;83(2) 357-372. doi: 10.1007/s00426-018-1066-8. Epub 2018 Aug 2. PubMed PMID: 30073406

13. Hanslmayr S, Axmacher N, Inman CS. Modulating Human Memory via Entrainment of Brain Oscillations. Trends Neurosci. 2019 Jul;42(7):485-499. doi: 10.1016/j.tins.2019.04.004. Epub 2019 Jun 6. Review. PubMed PMID: 31178076.

14. Hommel B, Sellaro R, Fischer R, Borg S, Colzato LS. High-Frequency Binaural Beats Increase Cognitive Flexibility: Evidence from Dual-Task Crosstalk. Front Psychol. 2016 Aug 24;7:1287. doi: 10.3389/fpsyg.2016.01287. eCollection 2016. PMID: 27605922 [PubMed].

15. Huang TL, Charyton C. A comprehensive review of the psychological effects of brainwave entrainment. Altern Ther Health Med. 2008 Sep-Oct;14(5):38-50. Review. Erratum in: Altern Ther Health Med. 2008 Nov-Dec;14(6):18. PubMed PMID: 18780583

16. Lane JD, Kasian SJ, Owens JE, Marsh GR. Binaural auditory beats affect vigilance performance and mood. Physiol Behav. 1998 Jan;63(2):249-52. PubMed PMID: 9423966.

17. Le Scouarnec RP, Poirier RM, Owens JE, Gauthier J, Taylor AG, Foresman PA. Use of binaural beat tapes for treatment of anxiety: a pilot study of tape preference and outcomes. Altern Ther Health Med. 2001 Jan;7(1):58-63. PMID: 11191043

18. Notbohm A, Herrmann CS. Flicker Regularity Is Crucial for Entrainment of Alpha Oscillations. Front Hum Neurosci. 2016 Oct 13;10:503. eCollection 2016. PubMed PMID: 27790105; PubMed Central PMCID: PMC5061822.

19. Oster, G. Auditory beats in the brain. Scientific American, 229, 94–102, 1973.

20. Padmanabhan R, Hildreth AJ, Laws D. A prospective, randomised, controlled study examining binaural beat audio and pre-operative anxiety in patients undergoing general anaesthesia for day case surgery. Anaesthesia. 2005 Sep;60(9):874-7. PMID: 16115248

21. Pandya PK, Krishnan A. Human frequency-following response correlates of the distortion product at 2F1-F2. J Am Acad Audiol. 2004 Mar;15(3):184-97. PubMed PMID: 15119460.

22. Radeloff A, Cebulla M, Shehata-Dieler W. [Auditory evoked potentials: basics and clinical applications]. Laryngorhinootologie. 2014 Sep;93(9):625-37. doi:10.1055/s-0034-1385868. Epub 2014 Aug 25. Review.

23. Reedijk SA, Bolders A, Hommel B. The impact of binaural beats on creativity. Front Hum Neurosci. 2013 Nov 14;7:786. doi: 10.3389/fnhum.2013.00786. eCollection 2013. PubMed PMID: 24294202; PubMed Central PMCID: PMC3827550.

24. Tang HY, Riegel B, McCurry SM, Vitiello MV. Open-Loop Audio-Visual Stimulation (AVS): A Useful Tool for Management of Insomnia? Appl Psychophysiol Biofeedback. 2016 Mar;41(1):39-46. doi: 10.1007/s10484-015-9308-7. Review. PubMed PMID: 26294268.

25. Tang HY, Vitiello MV, Perlis M, Riegel B. Open-Loop Neurofeedback Audiovisual Stimulation: A Pilot Study of Its Potential for Sleep Induction in Older Adults. Appl Psychophysiol Biofeedback. 2015 Sep;40(3):183-8. doi: 10.1007/s10484-015-9285-x. PubMed PMID: 25931250; PubMed Central PMCID: PMC4534306.

26. Tatum, W. Handbook of EEG interpretation (2nd ed.). New York: Demos Medical Publishing LLC, 2014.

27. Thompson, M., & Thompson, L. The neurofeedback book: An introduction to basic concepts in applied psychophysiology. Wheat Ridge, CO: The Association for Applied Psychophyiology and Biofeedback, 2003.

28. Thut G, Veniero D, Romei V, Miniussi C, Schyns P, Gross J. Rhythmic TMS causes local entrainment of natural oscillatory signatures. Curr Biol. 2011 Jul 26;21(14):1176-85. doi: 10.1016/j.cub.2011.05.049. Epub 2011 Jun 30. PubMed PMID: 21723129; PubMed Central PMCID: PMC3176892.

29. Timmermann DL, Lubar JF, Rasey HW, Frederick JA. Effects of 20-min audio-visual stimulation (AVS) at dominant alpha frequency and twice dominant alpha frequency on the cortical EEG. Int J Psychophysiol. 1999 Apr;32(1):55-61. PubMed PMID: 10192008.

30. Wahbeh H, Calabrese C, Zwickey H, Zajdel D. Binaural beat technology in humans: a pilot study to assess neuropsychologic, physiologic, and electroencephalographic effects. J Altern Complement Med. 2007b Mar;13(2):199-206. PMID: 17388762

31. Weiland TJ, Jelinek GA, Macarow KE, Samartzis P, Brown DM, Grierson EM, Winter C. Original sound compositions reduce anxiety in emergency department patients: a randomised controlled trial. Med J Aust. 2011 Dec 19;195(11-12):694-8. PMID: 22171868.

32. Zampi DD. Efficacy of Theta Binaural Beats for the Treatment of Chronic Pain. Altern Ther Health Med. 2016 Jan-Feb;22(1):32-8. PubMed PMID: 26773319.